国家卫生和计划生育委员会"十三五"规划教材

高等卫生职业教育应用技能型规划教材

供高等卫生职业教育各专业用

医 护 英 语

主 审 商亚珍

主 编 秦博文 刘清泉

副主编 罗晓冰 封育新 保 静 孙 燕

编 者（以姓氏笔画为序）

王 矗（大庆医学高等专科学校）

王利亚（安徽医学高等专科学校）

王蕊蕊（皖西卫生职业学院）

吕小君（承德护理职业学院）

刘清泉（黑龙江护理高等专科学校）

孙 燕（合肥职业技术学院）

孙延宁（山东医学高等专科学校）

纪敬敏（河北中医学院）

陈明慧（皖北卫生职业学院）

陈精华（安徽人口职业学院）

罗晓冰（承德护理职业学院）

封育新（廊坊卫生职业学院）

保 静（甘肃卫生职业学院）

秦博文（承德护理职业学院）

唐瑞娟（合肥职业技术学院）

人民卫生出版社

图书在版编目（CIP）数据

医护英语 / 秦博文, 刘清泉主编. —北京：人民卫生出版社，2016

ISBN 978-7-117-22647-9

Ⅰ. ①医… Ⅱ. ①秦… ②刘… Ⅲ. ①医学－英语－医学院校－教材 Ⅳ. ①R

中国版本图书馆 CIP 数据核字（2017）第 012164 号

| 人卫智网 | www.ipmph.com | 医学教育、学术、考试、健康，购书智慧智能综合服务平台 |
| 人卫官网 | www.pmph.com | 人卫官方资讯发布平台 |

医 护 英 语

主　　编：秦博文　刘清泉

出版发行：人民卫生出版社（中继线 010-59780011）

地　　址：北京市朝阳区潘家园南里 19 号

邮　　编：100021

E - mail：pmph @ pmph.com

购书热线：010-59787592　010-59787584　010-65264830

印　　刷：河北博文科技印务有限公司

经　　销：新华书店

开　　本：850×1168　1/16　印张：14

字　　数：376 千字

版　　次：2017 年 2 月第 1 版　2024 年 12 月第 1 版第 12 次印刷

标准书号：ISBN 978-7-117-22647-9/R·22648

定　　价：34.00 元

打击盗版举报电话：010-59787491　E-mail：WQ @ pmph.com
（凡属印装质量问题请与本社市场营销中心联系退换）

出 版 说 明

为全面落实教育规划纲要,贯彻《国务院关于加快发展现代职业教育的决定》精神,体现"以服务为宗旨,以就业为导向,以能力为本位"的人才培养模式,遵循应用技能型人才成长规律,积极落实卫生职业教育改革发展的最新成果,创新编写模式。2015 年 7 月全国卫生职业教育教材建设指导委员会、人民卫生出版社组织全国近 30 余所高等卫生职业院校,成立了高等卫生职业教育应用技能型规划教材评审委员会,规划并组织国内高等卫生职业教育领域教学一线及临床工作一线的优秀专家编写了本套高等卫生职业教育应用技能型规划教材。

本套教材特点如下:

1. **顺应需求,符合要求** 教材融传授知识、培养能力、提高技能、提升素质为一体,注重职业教育人才德能并重、知行合一和崇高职业精神的培养。重视培养学生的创新、获取信息及终身学习的能力。实现高职教材有机衔接与过渡作用,并将职业道德、人文素养教育贯穿培养全过程,为中高衔接、高本衔接的贯通人才培养通道做好准备。

2. **坚持品质,突出"技能"** 教材编写遵循"三基、五性、三特定"的编写原则,坚持人民卫生出版社高质量医药教材的一贯品质。教材规划定位于应用技能型教材,旨在体现专业价值的同时,内容和工作岗位需求紧密衔接,并在各课程教材中加强对学生人文素质的培养。整套教材以"早期接触临床,早期接触岗位,早期接触社会"为引导,编写队伍引入临床一线教师,力争实现教材内容与职业岗位能力要求对接零距离。

3. **"纸数融合",特色鲜明** 全套教材采用全新编写模式,以扫描二维码形式,帮助老师及学生在移动终端共享优质配套网络资源,实现纸媒教材与富媒体教材资源的融合;配套习题内容更贴近执业资格考试内容,实现移动终端同步答题与评测;为学生理解、巩固知识提供了全新的途径与独特的体验,全面体现"以学生为中心"的教材开发与建设理念。

高等卫生职业教育应用技能型规划教材首批共 44 种,将于 2016 年 9 月前陆续出版,供各卫生职业院校选用。

高等卫生职业教育应用技能型规划教材
目 录

序号	名称	主编	适用专业
1	护理伦理学基础	李 玲 杨金奎	护理、助产专业
2	卫生法律法规	苏碧芳 陈兰云	高等卫生职业教育各专业
3	体育与健康	周 非 邢 峰	高等卫生职业教育各专业
4	大学生心理健康	王江红 曹建琴	高等卫生职业教育各专业
5	护理礼仪与美学	袁慧玲 韩同敏	护理、助产专业
6	人际沟通	郑荣日 韩景新	高等卫生职业教育各专业
7	护理心理学基础	孙 萍 邓斌菊	护理、助产专业
8	医学生应用文写作	王劲松 冉隆平	高等卫生职业教育各专业
9	职业生涯规划与就业创业指导	潘传中 施向阳 蒋 伟	高等卫生职业教育各专业
10	计算机应用基础	章炳林 赵 娟	高等卫生职业教育各专业
11	医护英语	秦博文 刘清泉	高等卫生职业教育各专业
12	医用化学	段卫东 段广河	高等卫生职业教育各专业
13	正常人体结构	夏广军 隋月林	护理、助产专业
14	正常人体功能	彭 波 李桐楠	护理、助产专业
15	疾病学基础	夏广军 吴义春	护理、助产等相关专业
16	人体解剖学与组织胚胎学	任 晖 胡捍卫	护理、助产、临床医学等相关专业
17	生理学	杨桂染 周晓隆	护理、助产、临床医学等相关专业
18	生物化学	张又良 郭桂平	护理、助产、临床医学等相关专业
19	病理学与病理生理学	张军荣 李 夏	护理、助产、临床医学等相关专业
20	病原生物与免疫学	曹元应 曹德明	护理、助产、临床医学等相关专业
21	护理药理学	黄 刚 方士英	护理、助产专业
22	药理学	吴 艳 王迎新	临床医学、护理、助产等相关专业
23	健康评估	王新颖 杨 颖	护理、助产专业
24	护理学基础	程玉莲 余安汇	护理、助产专业
25	护理学导论	张琳琳 王慧玲	护理、助产专业
26	基础护理技术	周春美 陈焕芬	护理、助产专业
27	内科护理	马秀芬 王 婧	护理、助产专业
28	外科护理	郭书芹 王叙德	护理、助产专业
29	妇产科护理	李淑文 王丽君	护理专业
30	儿科护理	张玉兰 卢敏芳	护理、助产专业

续表

序号	名称	主编	适用专业
31	营养与膳食	林 杰 闫瑞霞	护理、助产专业
32	急危重症护理	狄树亭 万紫旭	护理、助产专业
33	中医护理	屈玉明 才晓茹	护理、助产专业
34	眼耳鼻喉口腔科护理	桂 平 张爱芳	护理、助产专业
35	传染病护理	吴惠珍 尤雪剑	护理、助产专业
36	精神科护理	王凤荣 马文华	护理、助产专业
37	社区护理	姜新峰 王秀清	护理、助产专业
38	老年护理	李玉明 郝 静	护理、助产专业
39	护理管理	周更苏 白建英	护理、助产专业
40	助产学	郭艳春 王玉蓉	助产专业
41	妇科护理	杨淑臻 郭雅静	助产专业
42	遗传与优生	王洪波 王敬红	护理、助产专业
43	母婴保健	王黎英	助产专业
44	护理技能综合实训	黄弋冰 卢玉彬	护理、助产专业

高等卫生职业教育应用技能型规划教材
评审委员会名单

顾　问

　　文历阳（华中科技大学同济医学院）　　杨文秀（天津医学高等专科学校）

主任委员

　　陈命家（安徽医学高等专科学校）

副主任委员

　　刘祁杰（忻州职业技术学院）　　杨金奎（安庆医药高等专科学校）

　　刘更新（廊坊卫生职业学院）　　周建军（重庆三峡医药高等专科学校）

　　秦国杰（临汾职业技术学院）　　王大成（乌兰察布医学高等专科学校）

执行委员会主任

　　彭　波（黑龙江护理高等专科学校）　　窦天舒（人民卫生出版社）

　　黄　刚（甘肃卫生职业学院）

执行委员会副主任

　　张玉兰（大庆医学高等专科学校）　　谭　工（重庆三峡医学高等专科学校）

　　邓　瑞（河西学院医学院）　　才晓茹（沧州医学高等专科学校）

　　屈玉明（山西职工医学院）

委　员（按姓氏笔画排序）

　　于彦章（临汾职业技术学院）　　张又良（安徽人口职业学院）

　　王长智（潍坊护理职业学院）　　张来平（陇东学院岐伯医学院）

　　王晓玲（陇东学院岐伯医学院）　　周晓隆（合肥职业技术学院）

　　方士英（皖西卫生职业学院）　　胡雪芬（大兴安岭职业学院）

　　马　莉（唐山职业技术学院）　　潘玉华（武威职业学院）

　　李朝鹏（邢台医学高等专科学校）　　潘传中（达州职业技术学院）

　　宋印利（哈尔滨医科大学大庆校区）

执行委员会委员（按姓氏笔画排序）

　　丁言华（大兴安岭职业学院）　　李　菊（临汾职业技术学院）

　　王万荣（安徽医学高等专科学校）　　李东禄（甘肃医学院）

　　朱小平（河西医学院）　　杨　颖（山西职工医学院）

　　孙　萍（重庆三峡医药高等专科学校）　　吴　艳（大庆医学高等专科学校）

　　周慧春（唐山职业技术学院）　　张开礼（武威职业学院）

　　李　夏（山西职工医学院）　　张军荣（甘肃卫生职业学院）

　　李　峰（皖西卫生职业学院）　　苑建兵（张家口学院护理学院）

林　杰（黑龙江护理高等专科学校）　　谈永进（安庆医药高等专科学校）

金玉忠（沧州医学高等专科学校）　　曹聪云（邢台医学高等专科学校）

郝　静（山西忻州职业技术学院）　　董会龙（菏泽家政职业学院）

段广河（廊坊卫生职业学院）　　　　程　琳（四川中医药高等专科学校）

秦爱军（河北中医学院护理学院）　　焦　烽（通辽职业学院）

桂　平（安徽人口职业学院）　　　　蔡　锋（哈尔滨医科大学大庆校区）

徐国辉（承德护理职业学院）

秘　书

张　峥（人民卫生出版社）

网络增值服务（数字配套教材）
编者名单

主　编　秦博文　刘清泉

副主编　吕小君　罗晓冰　封育新　保　静　孙　燕

编　者（以姓氏笔画为序）

王　矗（大庆医学高等专科学校）

王利亚（安徽医学高等专科学校）

王蕊蕊（皖西卫生职业学院）

吕小君（承德护理职业学院）

刘清泉（黑龙江护理高等专科学校）

孙　燕（合肥职业技术学院）

孙延宁（山东医学高等专科学校）

纪敬敏（河北中医学院）

陈明慧（皖北卫生职业学院）

陈精华（安徽人口职业学院）

罗晓冰（承德护理职业学院）

封育新（廊坊卫生职业学院）

保　静（甘肃卫生职业学院）

秦博文（承德护理职业学院）

唐瑞娟（合肥职业技术学院）

前　言

为深入贯彻《国务院关于加快发展现代职业教育的决定》，创新发展高等卫生职业教育，科学构建现代职业教育课程体系，培养职业素养与专业知识、专业技能并重的技能型卫生专门人才。经全国高等医药教材建设研究会和人民卫生出版社共同研究决定，启动新一轮高等卫生职业教育应用技能型规划教材编写工作。

本册《医护英语》教材遵从教育部对高等卫生职业教育的培养目标、结合高职医护专业学生的学习特点、以及《医护英护》学科的课程特色进行编写大纲的制定，以进一步适应医护人才国际化发展，满足国内外人才市场资源配置的需要。编写大纲制定之前主编进行了大量的调研工作：①调研全国部分省市的医护高职院校医护专业英语的教学情况（教材情况、任课教师情况、学生学习情况）；②收集并分析发达国家护士资格考试试题、分析不同国家应聘护士面试、口试试题的特点，将其考试精髓融入到本教材中；③收集并分析全国医护英语水平考试试题特点，并将其融入到本教材中。

《医护英语》不同于公共英语，是医护工作者在实施医护工作时应用的语言，它具有特定环境、特定语境等特点。因此，学生应具备与病人及家属交流的技能；能用英语书写护理记录、制定护理计划的能力。具备在工作中听、说、读、写全方面的能力，并能顺利通过国内医护英语考试和各种出国护士考试。

本着以上两大原则和目标，本教材进行如下编写：共设十二个单元，每单元分听、说、读、写、词汇扩展和补充练习六个部分。教材的内容选材以医院为主线，编写形式以病人就诊时医护人员的技能为主，分别为：出院和住院、护理技能、心血管科、呼吸科、消化科、血液、免疫和内分泌科，神经病科，泌尿生殖科，产科和妇科，儿科，老年病科以及外科。在词汇扩展部分，根据医学词汇的构词特点，采取词根和词缀相结合的记忆方法，方便学生能够更快更好地去掌握。在补充练习部分，选用近五年以来的出国护士培训真题，以便使学生能够掌握最新的出题模式和考试动向。此外，本书的另一个特点是根据李克强总理"互联网＋"的行动计划，推动信息技术与传统产业的生态结合，我们将纸质媒介与电子媒介相结合，增加了富媒体内容，使学生能够随时随地使用移动设备就可以学习书本上的内容。

本册《医护英语》教材由主编、副主编和编者们通力合作，经承德医学院商亚珍教授主审，出版社大力协助，得以出版面世，在此一并致以诚挚的感谢，教材在编写过程中难免有不妥之处，请各位专家及读者指正。

秦博文　刘清泉

2016 年 11 月

Content

Content

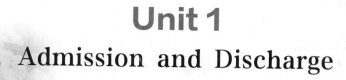

Unit 1
Admission and Discharge

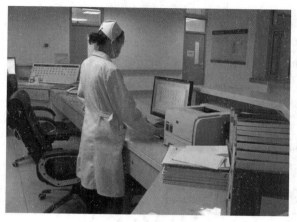

Fig. 1-1　nurse station

Cheerfulness is the promoter of health. 心情愉快是健康的增进剂。

——Joseph Addison（约瑟夫·艾迪生）

Learning Objectives

Skill focus

1. *Master the dialogues of "Admission and Discharge" and practice them with your partner.*
2. *Know the methods of the physical examination.*
3. *Understand how to collect the data of nursing assessment.*

Language focus

1. *Be familiar with the words, phrases related to "Admission and Discharge".*
2. *Be able to state the "Nursing Assessment" and "the Physical Examination".*

Part Ⅰ　Listening

　　This section is designed to test your ability to understand spoken English in the first visit or registration. You will hear a selection of recorded materials and you must answer the questions that accompany them. There are TWO parts in this section, Part A and Part B.

Part A

Words in Focus

symptom /ˈsimtəm, ˈsimp-/　　　　　　　　　*n.*　　　症状；征兆

ER-1-1
扫一扫 读一读

ER-1-2
扫一扫 看一看

笔记

register /ˈrɛdʒistə/	v.	登记；注册
insurance /inˈʃʊrəns/	n.	保险费；保险
claim /kleim/	v.	声称；索取
registration /ˌrɛdʒiˈstreiʃən/	n.	挂号；登记

Useful Expressions

the department of internal medicine	内科
health insurance	医疗保险
insurance company	保险公司

Text

ER-1-3
扫一扫 听一
听

ER-1-4
扫一扫 知情
节

Directions:

You're going to hear a short dialogue. Before listening, you will have 5 seconds to read each of the questions which accompany it. Listen to the dialogue and answer the following questions.

Background:

The following conversation is about the first visit. According to the Tony's symptoms, the nurse, Lily advises which department he should register with and tells where the Department of Internal Medicine is.

Comprehension of the text

1. What are the patient's symptoms?

   A. vomiting

   B. diarrhea

   C. temperature, tired and aching

2. Which department does the nurse advice Tony to register with?

   A. the department of internal medicine

   B. the emergency room

   C. not mentioned

3. What does the patient do before he leaves the hospital?

   A. see an internal medicine doctor

   B. pay his medical cost

   C. not mentioned

4. Does the patient have health insurance?

   A. no   B. yes   C. not mentioned

5. Where is the department of internal medicine?

   A. on the third floor   B. on the second floor   C. on the fourth floor

ER-1-5
扫一扫 读一
读

ER-1-6
扫一扫 看一
看

笔 记

Part B

Words in Focus

cough /kɔ:f/	n.	咳嗽
surgeon /ˈsɜːrdʒən/	n.	外科医生
file /fail/	n.	档案，文件
condition /kənˈdiʃən/	n.	状态；健康状况
physician /fiˈziʃən/	n.	内科医生

Useful Expressions

on file	存档
Consulting Room	诊室；诊疗室
Drug Store	药房

Text

ER-1-7
扫一扫 听一听

Directions: *In this section, you're going to hear a conversation three times. When the conversation is read for the first time, you should listen carefully for its general idea. When the conversation is read for the second time, you are required to fill in the blanks with the exact sentences or phrases you have just heard. Finally, when the conversation is read for the third time, you should check what you have written.*

Background:

  The following conversation is about registration.

Comprehension of the text

Nancy: What can I do for you?

Tom: I want to see a doctor. I don't feel very well, but I don't know what to do.

Nancy: What's the problem?

Tom: Since last night I have had a bad cough.

Nancy: _____.

Tom: Yes.

Nancy: _____.

Tom: Yes, I have one.

Nancy: Do you remember your card number?

Tom: No, I can't remember it.

Nancy: OK, no problem. _____.

Tom: Thank you.

Nancy: _____.

Tom: I want to_____.

Nancy: _____.

Tom: Oh, I see.

Nancy: This is your file. Please don't lose it, and remember to bring it whenever you come. Do you have any other questions?

Tom: Yes, _____.

Nancy: Go down this road until _____. Make a left turn and it is just there.

Tom: Thank you.

Nancy: You are welcome.

(265 words)

Part II　Speaking

  This section is designed to test your speaking ability. After learning the following conversation A and B you will have the ability of speaking skill in Admission and Discharging, try to do the following speaking tasks.

笔记

ER-1-9
扫一扫 听一听

ER-1-10
扫一扫 知情节

Conversation 1

Admission

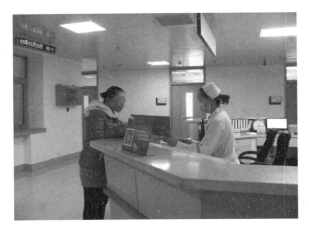

Fig. 1-2   admission

Background:

　　Mrs. Green comes to the ward. Joan is the head nurse of this department. Carrie introduces Dr. David to Mrs. Green and tells her how to use a nurse-call system. Carrie also answers some questions that Mrs. Green puts forward.

Joan: Welcome Mrs. Green. I'm the nurse in charge of this department. Please make yourself at home. Someone is now tidying up the patient-bed for you. You can check in at the reception desk and then have a rest in the waiting room.

Mrs. Green: Thank you. I'm sorry to trouble you so much.

Joan: Don't mention it. It's just our job.

After a while

Mrs. Green: Oh，it's a little honey room.

Carrie: I'm glad you like it.

Mrs. Green: Can I have your name?

Carrie: My name is Carrie. Welcome to our ward. Everything is ready.

Mrs. Green: Excuse me. Where is my bed?

Carrie: This way, please. Your bed is No. 202. The panel on the head of the bed is equipped with a nurse-call system. If you need anything, you can press this button. Each of the nurses will come as soon as possible.

Mrs. Green: It's very kind of you.

Carrie: Dr. David is responsible for your treatment. He is very kind and considerate. There are some very common exams that an inpatient must take, and there are some special examinations based on your disease. Dr. David will talk about it.

Mrs. Green: Oh, I got it.

Carrie: Dr. David is very good at the diagnosis and treatment on this kind of disease. I'm sure you will get a remarkable recovery. If you need anything, don't hesitate to let me know.

笔记

Mrs. Green:　Thanks. When will the morning ward round begin?

Carrie:　The ward round starts at 8:00 a.m. every morning.

Mrs. Green:　Will the nurse watch the patients at night?

Carrie:　Yes, the nurse on duty makes two rounds of the wards during the night.

Mrs. Green:　When are my relatives allowed to visit me?

Carrie:　The visiting hours are from 3:00 to 5: 00 p.m.

Mrs. Green:　Must I be confined to the ward?

Carrie:　Not exactly. You can go to the garden downstairs for a walk, but you must let us know.

Mrs. Green:　OK.

Carrie:　You can have a rest now. Dr. David will come to see you 20 minutes later.

Mrs. Green:　I'll be here waiting for him. See you later.

Carrie:　See you later.

(408 words)

Words in Focus

ward /wɔːrd/	n.	病房
responsible /riˈspɑːnsəbl/	adj.	负责任的；尽责的
treatment /ˈtriːtmənt/	n.	治疗；处理
considerate /kənˈsidərət/	adj.	体贴的；深思熟虑的
inpatient /ˈinˌpeiʃənt/	n.	住院病人
diagnosis /ˌdaiəɡˈnousis/	n.	诊断
recovery /riˈkʌvəri/	n.	恢复；复原
hesitate /ˈheziteit/	vi.	犹豫
relative /ˈrɛlətiv/	n.	亲属；亲戚
confine /kənˈfain/	vt.	限制；局限于

ER-1-11
扫一扫 读一读

ER-1-12
扫一扫 看一看

Useful Expressions

in charge of	负责；主管
tidy up	收拾
patient bed	病床
check in	登记
the reception desk	接待台

I. Free talk

Directions: Work in pairs and discuss the following questions after learning to recording of Dialogue One.

1. What kind of person is Dr. David?

_____

_____

2. Which regulation should Mrs. Green obey?

_____

_____

3. Must Mrs. Green be confined to the ward? What can she do?

_____

_____

笔记

II. Comprehension of the text

Directions: According to the following conversation, complete the sentences.

1. Mrs. Green can check in at _____ and then have a rest in the waiting room.

   A. registration   B. the information desk   C. the reception desk

2. If Mrs. Green needs anything, what should she do?

   A. press the button of a nurse-call system

   B. ask the nurse in person

   C. ask the ward mate to help

3. _____ that an inpatient must take.

   A. some special examinations

   B. nothing

   C. some very common examinations

4. How many times does the nurse watch the patient during the night?

   A. once   B. twice   C. none

5. When will the morning ward round begin?

   A. 8:00 a.m. every morning   B. from 8:00 to 10:00 a.m.   C. 8:30 a.m. every morning

Conversation 2

Discharging

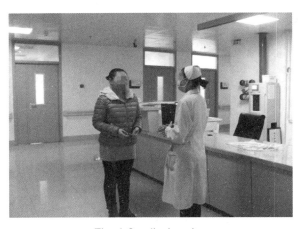

Fig. 1-3   discharging

Background:

Bruce will be discharged tomorrow. Nurse, named Tina, is giving him some suggestions.

Tina: Good morning, Bruce, you look so fresh.

Bruce: Morning, Tina. I really feel strong and fit.

Tina: I have good news to you.

Bruce: Really? What is it?

Tina: The doctor says that all the tests were normal. You are going to be discharged tomorrow. Congratulations!

Bruce: Is that so? I am so happy to hear that.

Tina: You have been in the hospital for two weeks, haven't you?

Bruce: Exactly, but Dr. David told me that I still have to rest for several weeks.

Tina: Dr. David has written the certificate for you.

Bruce: Could you give me some suggestions?

Tina: Er... Firstly, live a regular life and have a rest. Secondly, give up smoking and drinking. Have more nutritious food. Thirdly, don't stimulate the incision when you have a bath. Finally, come here to have an examination a month later.

Bruce: Thank you very much.

Tina: You are welcome.

Bruce: Do I need to continue taking medicine?

Tina: Yes, the doctor will prescribe some medicine for you.

Bruce: What medicine should I take?

Tina: Some antibiotic medicine.

Bruce: Where can I get?

Tina: The doctor will give you the prescription, and you will need to go the Pharmacy Department, I will show you how to get there tomorrow.

Bruce: Ok, will the doctor send a letter to my insurance company?

Tina: Sure. Also, the doctor will write a letter for your family doctor and explain the treatment you have received.

Bruce: Thanks a lot. Please give me the bill.

Tina: I will go to the Admission Office for it at once.

Bruce: Thank you. All the doctors and nurses here are very kind. I will always remember you.

Tina: It is our responsibility.

(301 words)

Words in Focus

discharge /dis'tʃɑːdʒ/	vi./n.	出院
certificate /sə'tifikit/	n.	证明书
regular /'regjulə/	adj.	有规律的；定期的；经常的
stimulate /'stimjuleit/	vt.	刺激；激励
incision /in'siʒən/	n.	切开；切口
nutritious /njuː'triʃəs/	adj.	有营养的；滋养的
prescribe /pri'skraib/	vi.	开处方
antibiotic /ˌæntibaɪ'ɔtik/	n.	抗生素
pharmacy /'fɑːməsi/	n.	药房

ER-1-16
扫一扫 读一读

Useful Expressions

Admission Office   住院处

ER-1-17
扫一扫 看一看

I. Free talk

Directions: *Work in pairs and discuss the following questions after learning to the Dialogue Two.*

1. How many suggestions does Tina give Bruce?

_____

_____

2. What are three suggestions that Tina gives Bruce?

_____

_____

笔记

3. What will the doctor give Bruce?

_____

_____

II. Comprehension of the Text

Directions: *According to the following conversation and complete the sentences.*

1. How long did Bruce stay in the hospital?

   A. three weeks   B. two weeks   C. don't mention it

2. What will Bruce give up?

   A. smoking   B. smoking and drinking   C. drinking

3. When will Bruce need to come back to have an examination?

   A. a month later   B. in two weeks   C. don't mention it

4. What medicine should Bruce take?

   A. the painkillers   B. some antibiotic medicine   C. don't mention it

5. Where will Tina go to for the bill?

   A. pharmacy department   B. insurance company   C. admission office

Part Ⅲ   Reading

Text A

> Nursing assessment is the first and most critical step of nursing process. Nurses collect the information which requires writing a patient's diagnoses and care plan by communicating with the patient or others, observing the patient's reactions and taking vital signs.
>
> **Pre-reading**
> 1. What is the process of nursing assessment?
> 2. What is the purpose of nursing assessment?

Nursing Assessment

The nursing assessment, the first step in delivering nursing care, is an organized and dynamic process. The process of the nursing assessment involves two parts: one is collecting and organizing the data; The other is documenting and analyzing the data. Data is classified as either objective or subjective. Subjective data refers to "symptoms" that the patient describes, and it can also be obtained from the family, significant others, health care team members and health records. Objective data are the signs that can be observed, measured and verified.

The purpose of the nursing assessment is to establish a database. The relevant information is collected including the patient's history (allergies, past surgeries, chronic disease, use of folk healing methods); physiological, psychological,

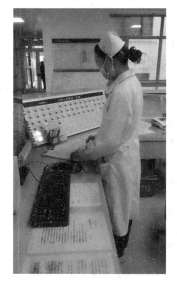

Fig. 1-4   nursing assessment

笔记

economic, socio-cultural, spiritual, and lifestyle factors that may affect patient's health status; current problems of patient (pain, nausea, sleep pattern, religious practices, medication or treatment the patient is taking now). The information contained in the database is the basis for developing nursing diagnosis and planning individualized nursing care.

A nurse uses every approach available to collect the information which requires writing a patient's diagnoses and care plan.

Communication with the patient or others　The patient himself is one of the most important assessment object in nursing process. A nurse carries out an initial detailed interview to get a full picture of the patient's physical and mental status by communicating with himself or his relatives. A nurse also makes shorter interviews throughout the day by asking the patient how he is feeling and other questions about his well-being. Communicating with other health care professionals involved in a patient's care is vital to assessment, especially when a patient is transferred from another location. In a hospital setting, a patient may be seen by a doctor, nurse, respiratory therapist, physical therapist or other specialists.

Observing the patient's reactions　Nurses use every interaction with patients as a way to gather information by observing the patient's responses to stimuli. This helps a nurse recognize the pain, emotional disturbances and reaction to treatment. It is an especially important approach for patients who are in no position to communicate.

Taking vital signs　The nurse should perform a head to toe assessment. Regular monitoring of a patient's heart rate, blood pressure, temperature and respiratory rate allows the nurse to help prevent fatal complications and evaluate a patient's overall condition.

Nursing assessment is the first and most critical step of nursing process. Accuracy of assessment data affects all other phases of the nursing process. A complete database allows the nurse to formulate nursing diagnosis and intervenes to promote to health and prevent disease.

(450 words)

Words in Focus

assessment /əˈsɛsmənt/	n.	评估；评价
dynamic /daiˈnæmik/	adj.	动态的；不断变化的
objective /əbˈdʒɛktiv/	adj.	客观的；目标的
subjective /səbˈdʒɛktiv/	adj.	主观的；个人的
relevant /ˈrɛlivənt/	adj.	有关的；相关联的
chronic /ˈkrɒnik/	adj.	慢性的；长期的
available /əˈveiləbə/	adj.	可获得的；有空的
initial /iˈniʃəl/	adj.	最初的；开始的
status /ˈsteitəs/	n.	情形；状态
respiratory /risˈpairətəri/ri'spirətəri/	adj.	呼吸的
observe /əbˈzɜːv/	v.	观察
response /riˈspɒns/	n.	反应；回答
stimuli /ˈstimjulai/	n.	刺激；刺激物
disturbance /diˈstɜːbəns/	n.	困扰；打扰
fatal /ˈfeitl/	adj.	致命的
complication /ˌkɒmpliˈkeiʃn/	n.	并发症

ER-1-21
扫一扫 读一读

ER-1-22
扫一扫 看一看

笔记

evaluate /iˈvæljuˌeit/	*vt.*	评价；对……评价
intervene /ˌintərˈviːn/	*vi.*	干预；阻碍

Useful Expressions

heart rate	心率（律）
blood pressure	血压
in no position to do	不能，不能够

Post-reading

I. Comprehension of the text

Choose the best answer to complete each sentence with the information from the text.

1. In delivering nursing care, _____ is the first step.
   A. assessment   B. treatment   C. diagnose

2. The purpose of the nursing assessment is to establish a _____.
   A. the patient's history   B. patient's health status   C. database

3. One of the most important assessment approaches in nursing process is _____.
   A. the patient herself   B. assessment   C. monitor

4. _____ is an especially important tool for patients who are in no position to communicate.
   A. communication   B. vital signs   C. observation

5. A(n) _____ database allows the nurse to formulate nursing diagnosis, develop client goals and intervenes to promote to health and prevent disease.
   A. accuracy   B. complete   C. initial

II. Vocabulary Activities

Find a word or phrase from the box below to complete each sentence. Change word forms where necessary.

assessment	available	status	respiratory	fatal
dynamic	initial	stimuli	disturbance	in no position to

1. The nursing assessment, the first step in delivering nursing care, is an organized and _____ process.

2. Observing helps a nurse recognizes the pain, emotional _____ and reaction to treatment.

3. A patient's chart provides information about his health _____.

4. In a hospital setting, a patient may be seen by a doctor, nurse, _____ therapist, physical therapist or other specialists.

5. A nurse carries out an _____ detailed interview to get a full picture of the patient's physical and mental status.

6. A nurse uses every tool _____ to collect the information which requires to write a patient's diagnoses and care plan.

7. Nurses use every interaction with patients as a way to gather information by observing the patients' responses to _____.

8. The patient herself is one of the most important _____ tools in nursing process.

9. It is an especially important tool for patients who are _____ communicate.

10. Regular monitoring of a patient's heart rate, blood pressure, temperature and respiratory rate allows the nurse to help prevent _____ complications and evaluate a patient's overall condition.

ER-1-23
扫一扫 答案
"晓"

ER-1-24
扫一扫 练一练

笔记

III. Supplementary

Text B

A physical examination is a routine test. For adults, we should have the physical examination at least once a year. There are four cardinal methods that can be performed during the physical examination.

Pre-reading

1. What is the first step in examining a patient?
2. Which aspects will the PCP also check?

ER-1-25
扫一扫 听一听

ER-1-26
扫一扫 知情节

Physical Examination

A physical examination is a routine test to check a person's overall health and make sure the body doesn't have any medical problems. The examination is also known as a wellness check. At abroad, the test should be performed by the primary care provider (PCP). A PCP may be a doctor, a nurse practitioner, or a physician assistant.

It is important that a person get a full physical examination at least once a year to notice any changes in our health status. All adults should have a yearly physical exam, especially in people over the age of 50, even if there are no existing health concerns. A physical examination not only helps the PCP to determine the general status of our health, but also gives us the opportunity to talk to the PCP about our physical or mental health concerns.

There are four cardinal methods that can be performed during the physical examination.

Inspection, the first step in examining a patient or body, is the search for any unusual marks or growths by observing the patient with PCP's eyes and sense of smell.

Palpation is employed on every part of the body accessible to the examining fingers. The PCP touches and feels the patient's body part with his hands to examine the consistency, location, size, tenderness, and texture of our individual organs.

Auscultation is a method used to "listen" the sounds of the body. The PCP will use the stethoscope to listen the person's heart or lungs to make sure there are no abnormal sounds.

Percussion is the act of striking the surface of the body to elicit a sound. This technique helps the PCP detect diaphragmatic movement, the size of heart, edge of liver and spleen.

The PCP will also check the person's temperature, respirations, blood pressure, height, weight, pulse and the lymph nodes.

Be sure to communicate with the PCP if we have any concerns throughout the exam. If we don't understand any test that our PCP is doing, don't hesitate to ask questions.

The PCP may be in touch with us after the exam. They will generally provide us with a copy of our test results. They will point out any problem areas and tell us anything that we should be doing. Depending on what our PCP finds, we may need other tests or screening at a later date. If no additional tests are needed and no health problems arise, we are set until next year.

(426 words)

Words in Focus

routine /ruːˈtiːn/   *adj.*   常规的；例行的

笔记

cardinal /ˈkɑːdinl/	adj.	基本的；最重要的
inspect /inˈspɛkt/	v.	检查；视察
palpation /pælˈpeiʃn/	n.	触诊
consistency /kənˈsistənsi/	n.	浓度；一致性
tenderness /ˈtɛndənis/	n.	触痛，压痛
texture /ˈtɛkstʃə/	n.	质地；纹理
auscultation /ˌɔskəlˈteiʃ ən/	n.	听诊
stethoscope /ˈsteθəskoʊp/	n.	听诊器
percussion /pəˈkʌʃn/	n.	叩诊
elicit /iˈlisit/	vt.	引起；引出
diaphragmatic /daiəfrægˈmætik/	adj.	横膈膜的

Useful Expressions

lymph nodes　　　　　　　　　　　淋巴结

Post-reading

I. Comprehension of the text

Choose the best answer to complete each sentence with the information from the text.

1. How often should we get a full physical examination?

   A. at least once a year　　　B. once two years　　　C. not mentioned

2. How many methods can be performed during the physical examination?

   A. five　　　　　　　　　B. four　　　　　　　C. three

3. Which method is the first step in examining a patient or body?

   A. percussion　　　　　　B. inspection　　　　　C. auscultation

4. The PCP will use the stethoscope to listen the person's heart or lungs. What is the method?

   A. percussion　　　　　　B. palpation　　　　　C. auscultation

5. Which method helps the PCP detect diaphragmatic movement, the size of heart, edge of liver and spleen?

   A. percussion　　　　　　B. palpation　　　　　C. auscultation

II. Vocabulary activities

Find a word or phrase from the box below to complete each sentence. Change word forms where is necessary.

| tenderness | routine | auscultation | stethoscope | inspect |
| palpation | percussion | diaphragmatic | cardinal | consistency |

1. The PCP touches and feels the patient's body part with his hands to examine the _____, location, size, _____, and texture of our individual organs.

2. _____ is a method used to "listen" the sounds of the body.

3. This technique helps the PCP detect _____ movement, the size of heart, edge of liver and spleen.

4. _____ is employed on every part of the body accessible to the examining fingers.

5. A physical examination is a _____ test to check a person's overall health and make sure the body doesn't have any medical problems.

6. The PCP will use the _____ to listen the person's heart or lungs to make sure there are no abnormal sounds.

笔记

7. _____ is the act of striking the surface of the body to elicit a sound.

8. _____ is the first step in examining a patient or body.

9. There are four _____ methods that can be performed during the physical exam.

III. Supplementary

ER-1-29
扫一扫 答案
"晓"

Part Ⅳ   Writing

Writing a Poster

ER-1-30
扫一扫 练一
练

Instructions:

A poster is any piece of printed paper designed to the attached to a wall or vertical surface. Typically posters include bots textual and graphic elements, although a poster may be are designed to be both eye-catching and informative.

Posters may be used for many purposes. They are a frequent tool of advertisers (particularly of events, musicians and films, propagandists, protesters and other groups trying to communicate a message.

Structure

A poster usually consists of the following parts:

1. the heading (Poster)

2. the body (the main content of the Poster)

3. the signature (organizer)

Examples

学术海报

题　目：如何处理医患关系

主讲人：赵××教授

时　间：4月14日（星期三）13:30—16:30

地　点：三楼学术报告厅

希望所有教师参加！

学院学术委员会

2005 年 4 月 10 日

Academic Lecture Poster

Topic: How to Deal with the Relationship between the Patient and the Doctor

Speaker: Prof. Zhao

Time: from13:30 to 16:30 on Thursday, April 14

Place: Academic Report Hall on the third floor

All teachers are expected to attend the lecture.

The College Academic Commission

April 10, 2005

Practice:

You are required to write a Poster according to the following instruction given in Chinese.

笔 记

13

说明：假设你是某医学院科研处的工作人员。学院将举办一次关于中医养生的学术讲座，本次讲座由科研处承办。请用英语书写一则海报。

_____

_____

_____

_____

_____

_____

_____

_____

ER-1-31
扫一扫 答案
"晓"

Part Ⅴ Enriching your word power

registration office	挂号处
out-patient department	门诊部
in-patient department	住院部
nursing department	护理部
emergency room	急诊室
admitting office	住院处
X-ray department/department of radiology	放射科
blood bank	血库
dispensary; pharmacy	药房
nutrition department	营养部
diet-preparation department	配膳室
therapeutic department	治疗室
disinfection-room	消毒室
dressing room	换药室
record room	病案室
doctor's office	医生办公室
nurses office	护士办公室
ward	病房
medical ward	内科病房
surgical ward	外科病房
pediatric ward	儿科病房
operation room (OR)	手术室
coronary care unit (CCU)	心脏重症室
intensive care unit (ICU)	重症室
neonatal intensive care unit (NICU)	新生儿重症室
medical department/department of internal medicine	内科
surgical department/department of surgery	外科
pediatrics department	小儿科
obstetrics and gynecology department	妇产科

笔记

labor room	待产室
delivery room	分娩室
ophthalmology department	眼科
dental department	牙科
ENT(ear-nose-throat) department	耳鼻喉科
urology department	泌尿科
dermatology department	皮肤科
plastic surgery	整形外科
anesthesiology department	麻醉科
pathology department	病理科
cardiology department	心脏病科
psychiatry department	精神病科
orthopedics department	骨科
neurology department	神经科
department of traditional Chinese medicine	中医科
department of infectious diseases	传染病科
geriatrics department	老人病专科
hematology department	血液科
hepatology department	肝病专科
nephrology department	肾脏科
department of physiotherapy	理疗科
electrotherapy room	电疗科
heliotherapy room	光疗科
wax-therapy room	蜡疗科
hydrotherapy room	水疗科
central laboratory	中心实验室
clinical laboratory	临床实验室
bacteriological laboratory	细菌实验室
biochemical laboratory	生化实验室
isolation room	隔离室

Part VI Exercise

Directions: *In this section, only one of the following options is correct, please choose.*

（王　蠹　秦博文）

ER-1-32
扫一扫 看一看

笔 记

Unit 2
Nursing Skills

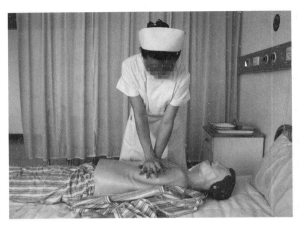

Fig. 2-1 nursing skills

Drunkenness is temporary suicide. 喝醉是暂时性的自杀。

——（Bertrand Russell（英国哲学家罗素）

Learning Objectives

Skill focus

1. *Master the routes of administration and nursing diagnosis.*
2. *Know how to apply the nursing process for clients.*
3. *Understand the overview on CPR.*

Language focus

1. *Master the language used in the relative clinic setting.*
2. *Learn the method of communication skills with patient.*

Part I Listening

This section is designed to test your ability to understand spoken English in nursing or medical contexts. You will hear a selection of recorded materials and you must answer the questions that accompany them. There are TWO parts in this section, Part A and Part B.

Part A

Words in Focus

systematic /ˌsɪstəˈmætɪk/	*adj.*	系统的；有条不紊的
framework /ˈfreɪmwɜːk/	*n.*	构架；框架

ER-2-1
扫一扫 读一读

ER-2-2
扫一扫 看一看

笔记

implementation /ˌɪmplɪmenˈteɪʃən/	n.	实施；贯彻；执行
measurable /ˈmeʒərəbəl/	adj.	可量度的；可测量的
document /ˈdɔːkjumənt/	v.	记录；证明
continuity /ˌkɔːntiˈnjuːiti/	n.	连续性；连贯；不间断
effectiveness /əˈfektivnis/	n.	作用；效应；效果
regression /riˈgreʃən/	n.	回到从前；回归；衰退

Useful Expressions

| set out | | 制定出；开始 |

Text

ER-2-3
扫一扫 听一
听

Directions: *In this section you will hear a short passage, at the end of the passage, one or more questions will be asked about what was said, decide which the best answer is.*

Background:

　　Whether you are working at the beginning of your career, or practicing at an advanced or specialist level, no matter what is your major. To be effective in nursing work, we must implement the steps of the nursing process. So what is nursing process?

Comprehension of the text

1. The nursing process begins with the step of _____.

   A. assessment　　　　　B. evaluation　　　　　C. implementation

2. Which step is the nurse's clinical judgment of the client's actual or potential condition?

   A. assessment　　　　　B. diagnosis　　　　　C. planning

ER-2-4
扫一扫 知情
节

3. According to the passage, which of the following statements is true?

   A. The nursing progress involves five major steps.

   B. Implementation is done according to the nurse's assessment.

   C. If progress towards the goal is slow, the nurse doesn't need to change the plan of care accordingly.

4. Is informed diagnosis important according to the passage?

   A. no　　　　　B. yes　　　　　C. not mentioned

5. The key point of the passage is that?

   A. How to write a nursing planning?

   B. The nursing progress involves five major steps.

   C. What is the nursing process?

Part B

Words in Focus

occupation /ˌɔːkjuˈpeiʃn/	n.	职业；工作
kindergarten /ˈkindəgɑːtn/	n.	幼儿园；学前班
pavement /ˈpeivmənt/	n.	人行道；硬路面
trip /trip/	v.	绊倒；绊
twist /twist/	v.	扭曲；扭转
swollen /ˈswəulən/	adj.	膨胀的；肿起的
orthopedist /ɔːθəuˈpiːdist/	n.	骨科医生；整形外科医师

ER-2-5
扫一扫 读一
读

ER-2-6
扫一扫 看一
看

Text

Directions: *You're going to hear one conversation. Before listening, you will have 5 seconds to*

笔记

17

ER-2-7
扫一扫 听一听

ER-2-8
扫一扫 知情节

read each of the questions that accompany it. While listening, answer each question by choosing A, B, or C. After listening, you will have 5 seconds to check your answer to each question.

Background:

　　Mr. Parkinson has tripped over on the pavement and twisted one of his ankles, which is swollen and very painful. So he decides to see a doctor. It's his first time to go the hospital. What will he do first? The following conversation is about registration, listen to it carefully and choose the right answer to each question.

Comprehension of the Text

1. Mr. Parkinson, have dizziness and sick.

　　A. yes　　　　　　　　B. no　　　　　　　　C. not mentioned

2. How old is Mr. Parkinson?

　　A. fifty-five years old　　B. forty-five years old　　C. forty-four years old

3. Which department does Mr. Parkinson want to register with?

　　A. orthopedist　　　　　B. oculist　　　　　　C. dentist

4. According to the dialogue, where is the Registrar Room?

　　A. on the third floor, on the right side of the stairs

　　B. on the third floor, on the left side of the stairs

　　C. on the second floor, on the left side of the stairs

5. According to the passage, which of the following statements is true?

　　A. Mr. Parkinson is an artist.

　　B. Mr. Parkinson will take an X-ray examination.

　　C. It's Mr. Parkinson's Second time to see the doctor.

Part Ⅱ　Speaking

　　This section is designed to test your speaking ability. After learning the following conversation A and B you will have the ability of speaking skill in medical and nursing working and try to do the following speaking tasks.

Conversation 1

Elimination

　　Mrs. Zhang has been in hospital for treatment of unstable angina. The nurse tells her to use a commode by the bed in order to reduce exertion and reduce the oxygen consumption. Mrs. Zhang tells the nurse that she has some difficulty in her bed. She can't go to the toilet in time and wet herself. She can't do things like normal people. What will the nurse do to help Mrs. Zhang?

Nurse:	Mrs. Zhang, what can I do for you?
Patient:	I think it's embarrassing to tell you that I can't hold on and I leak urine, and it does happen at different times. I need to pass water so often, but sometimes I don't make it in time and wet myself. Sometimes when I cough and laugh then the leaking happens.
Nurse:	How often do you pass urine?
Patient:	During the day it happens every two hours or so. It is bad at night. I frequently get out of bed to urinate. Always twice a night or more.

ER-2-9
扫一扫 听一听

ER-2-10
扫一扫 知情节

笔记

Nurse:	When did that happen?
Patient:	It may be about 3 years ago.
Nurse:	Have you told your General Practitioner when it happened?
Patient:	No, I don't know how to say, you know I think it's so embarrassing to tell someone else. Worse of all, I can't do things like normal people.
Nurse:	I'm sorry to hear that. But I think it's a common phenomenon in people similar to you. Don't worry about it because it may be successfully treated. How do you usually cope with the problem?
Patient:	At home, I try my best to go toilet, but most time I can't manage, I have plenty of washing to do. It is very difficult outside. If I need to pass urine I can't find a public toilet immediately. So I wear a paper diaper to cope with the leaks.
Nurse:	I will remember them and will add all these to your care plan then everyone knows your condition. If you need to spend a penny, everyone knows to bring the commode as soon as you need.
Patient:	OK, thank you!
Nurse:	When your angina has settled down, I will arrange for the nurse specialist to come to see you. She will do assessment and suggest ways that will improve your situation.
Patient:	Thank you!
Nurse:	Now I want to have a specimen of your urine to test that if you have an infection.
Patient:	I have to pee into a pot?
Nurse:	Yes, it is. But we only need the middle of the urine, not the urine that comes out first.
Patient:	OK.
Nurse:	Have you noticed any blood in your urine or an unusual smell?
Patient:	No.
Nurse:	Do you have any pain when you pass urine? Does it sting or burn?
Patient:	Never.
Nurse:	We need to have your information such as how often do you pass urine and the amount of your urine, and the amount of fluid intake.
Patient:	OK, and you will tell the nurses about how urgent it is when I want to pee.
Nurse:	Yes, of course I will. I'm putting it on the care plan, and I will tell the nurse who takes over from me. Can you think you could give me that sample now?
Patient:	Yes.
Nurse:	Do you have any other questions before I leave?
Patient:	No, I'm looking forward to seeing the experts.

(494 words)

Words in Focus

angina /ænˈdʒainə/	n.	心绞痛
commode /kəˈmoud/	n.	便桶；有抽屉的小柜
exertion /igˈzɜːʃn/	n.	费力；劳累
oxygen /ˈɔːksidʒən/	n.	氧；氧气
consumption /kənˈsʌmpʃən/	n.	消费；肺病；耗尽
urinate /ˈjuərineit/	v.	排尿；撒尿

ER-2-11
扫一扫 读一读

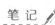

笔记

ER-2-12
扫一扫 看一看

phenomenon /fiˈnɑːminən/	*n.*	现象；事件
specimen /ˈspesimin/	*n.*	抽样；样品
sting /stiŋ/	*n.*	剧痛
burn /bɜːn/	*n.*	烧灼疼

Useful Expressions

hold on	坚持，固守
pass water	小便，排尿；小解
general practitioner	全科医师
paper diaper	纸尿裤
spend a penny	上厕所
settle down	安静下来；平息
nurse specialist	护理专家；专科护士

I. Free talk

Directions: Work in pairs and discuss the following questions after learning to the recording of Dialogue One.

1. Explain to your partner how does Mrs. Zhang usually cope with the problem?

_____

_____

_____

2. What are the problems of Mrs. Zhang?

_____

_____

_____

ER-2-13
扫一扫 答案
"晓"

ER-2-14
扫一扫 听一听

ER-2-15
扫一扫 知情节

笔记

II. Comprehension of the text

Directions: According to the following conversation and complete the sentences.

1. Mrs. Zhang thinks it's so _____ to tell somebody else.

   A. embarrassing   B. embarrassed   C. difficult

2. Mrs. Zhang thinks it is very difficult outside to pass urine because she can't find a public toilet _____.

   A. nearby   B. rapidly   C. immediately

3. The nurse adds all her condition to the care plan, so the patient need to _____, the nurses bring the commode to her.

   A. spending a penny   B. passing urine   C. pee

4. _____ is the nursing expert who can provide advanced care measures to improve the patient situation.

   A. Nursing Staff   B. Nurse Specialist   C. Senior Nurse

5. The nurse tells the patient if her angina has _____, she will tell the Nurse Specialist to help her for her illness.

   A. settled up   B. settled back   C. settled down

Conversation 2

Intravenous Infusion

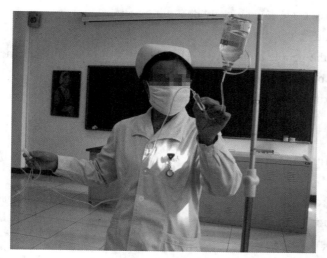

Fig. 2-2   Ⅳ infusion

The patient worries that the fluids is not effective, and the disease will not be recovered, so she does not want to be given injection. What should the nurse do to help the patient?

Nurse:　　Good morning, Mrs. Liu. I'm your nurse. Can I see your ID bracelet?

Patient:　　Sure.

Nurse:　　How are you feeling today?

Patient:　　Better.

Nurse:　　It's time for me to give you Ⅳ fluids. Show me your hand please.

Patient:　　OK.

Nurse:　　The Ⅳ time is a bit longer, if you need to go to the toilet please.

Patient:　　I just went to the bathroom. Thank you. Could you tell me about the purpose of the Ⅳ fluids?

Nurse:　　Of course. The fluids can provide water for your body and provide energy for your heart function. I will insert the needle, please make a fist.

Patient:　　OK. I think my heart is in a good condition, so can you let the fluid drop more quickly?

Nurse:　　I know your heart is in good condition. According to your state, age and the character of drugs to adjust the number of drops. The injection rate has been adjusted. Please do not change it. Your Ⅳ fluids must be given slowly so as not to overload you.

Patient:　　Well, I will follow you. But I think it's no use for me. So I don't need the injection any more.

Nurse:　　Don't get disheartened. You will soon recover after the treatment.

Patient:　　Perhaps you're right, but I always feel anxious. I think I'm a heavy burden on others.

Nurse:　　Mrs. Liu, you know we all care for you, especially your husband and children. Do what you're told. You can live a full, useful, and happy life.

笔记

21

Patient: No, I feel that everything in the world is meaningless. So I don't want to live in the world to bother others.

Nurse: Mrs. Liu, everyone has his own trouble, but he shouldn't see the world through dark-color glasses. He can correctly deal with matters.

Patient: Thank you.

Nurse: Look at the people around you. They are all full of confidence, never give up. I think you will be better soon.

Patient: Nice talking to you, I'm fine, please give me the injection.

(370 words)

Words in Focus

transfusion /træns'fjuʒən/	*n.*	输液；渗透
fist /fist/	*n.*	拳，拳头
arbitrarily /ˌɑbə'trɛrəli/	*adv.*	任意地；武断地
overload /ˌouvə'ləud/	*n.*	过多，过量；超负荷
dishearten /dis'hɑːtn/	*v.*	使失去勇气，使失去信心
embarrassing /im'bærəsiŋ/	*adj.*	使人尴尬的
shot /ʃɑt/	*n.*	注射；发射

I. Free talk

Directions: *Work in pairs and discuss the following questions after learning to the Dialogue Two*

1. What is the woman worried about?

_____

_____

2. Why does the nurse tell the patient that she can't adjust the fluid to drop more quickly?

_____

_____

3. How to communicate with the patients who appears psychological problems?

_____

_____

4. How to adjust the rate of fluid?

According to the patient's _____ , _____ , the _____ of drugs to adjust the number of drops, the general adult' 40～60 drops per minute; children's 20～40 drops per minute.

II. Conversation

Directions: *If you are a nurse to give an injection for a patient with fever, what should you tell to the patient about the injection before operating?*

_____

_____

笔记

Part Ⅲ　Reading

Text A

ER-2-19
扫一扫 听一听

ER-2-20
扫一扫 知情节

Many people in the world suffer cardiac arrest outside hospital every year. Some cardiac arrests happen in a private residential setting, and others happen in a public place. However, only a few of them can survive. Why? People simply do not know what to do? Would you know how to do if you find someone that had a cardiac arrest?

Pre-reading

1. Where is the location of the heart?
2. How to open the airway?

Cardiopulmonary Resuscitation(CPR)

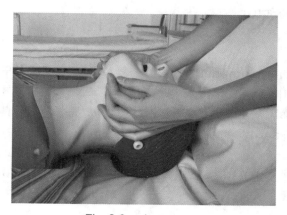

Fig. 2-3　airway open

Cardiopulmonary resuscitation is a lifesaving technique useful in many emergencies. Today it's such a lifesaving skill that is simple enough for anyone to learn. The steps of CPR are summarized by the CAB (Compressions, Airway and Breathing) to help the people remember the order to perform the steps of CPR.

Rescuing steps:

1. Check for danger: First, make sure that there are no hazards to the rescuer, the collapsed person or any other people nearby.

2. Check the patient's consciousness: Squeeze the person's shoulder firmly and say loudly "Are you OK?" If the person does not respond to you, send for help. Ask someone to call 120 or the local emergency number, someone to get an AED, the rescuer begins CPR.

3. Locate the person: Put the person on his or her back on a firm surface, such as the floor or a CPR board. If the person is in bed, place a back board under the client.

4. Initiate chest compressions: The pulse should be checked by palpating the carotid artery on one side of the neck for 5~10s. If no pulse is palpated, chest compressions should be initiated. Place the heel of one hand on the center of the chest. Place the other hand on top of the first hand. Meanwhile, keep your elbows straight and position your shoulders directly

笔记

above your hands. Push hard and fast on the center of the chest. The adult sternum should be depressed at least 2 inches (5cm). The rescuer should perform 30 compressions at a rate of at least 100 Per Minute.

5. Open the airway: First check the airway, open the person's mouth and look inside, clear the mouth of loose matter, such as food or denture. Then airway should be opened with a head-tilt, chin-lift maneuver. To perform this, place one hand on the person's forehead and press backward in a firm way. Lift the chin forward with fingers of the other hand. If neck injury is suspected, use the jaw thrust maneuver. To perform this, grasp the angles of the client's lower jaw and lift with both hands, one on each side.

6. Breathe for the person: Make sure the airway opened, cover his open mouth with your mouth, pinch his nose with your finger and thumb. Give 2 rescue breaths, and take about one second to complete each breath.

Thirty chests compressions followed by two rescue breaths are considered one cycle. You need to do five cycles. (About two minutes). Then check the client's carotid pulse and breathing. If the person has not begun to move or respond, continue CPR until there are signs of movement or ambulance paramedics arrive.

(449 words)

Words in Focus

ER-2-21
扫一扫 读一
读

ER-2-22
扫一扫 看一
看

cardiopulmonary /ˌkɑːdioʊˈpʌlmənəri/	adj.	心肺的
resuscitation /riˌsʌsiˈteiʃən/	n.	恢复知觉；苏醒
emergency /iˈmɜːdʒənsi/	n.	紧急情况；突发事件；急症
compression /kəmˈprɛʃən/	n.	压缩；压紧
collapse /kəˈlæps/	v.	倒塌；崩溃
conscious /ˈkɑːnʃəs/	adj.	有意识的；神志清醒的
squeeze /skwiːz/	v.	压缩；压迫
palpate /pælˈpeit/	v.	触诊
sternum /ˈstɜːnəm/	n.	胸骨；胸片
pinch /pintʃ/	v.	捏；挤痛
carotid /kəˈrɑtid/	adj.	颈动脉的

Useful Expressions

AED (automated external defibrillator)	体外自动除颤器
chin-lift	抬头举颏法
jaw thrust maneuver	双手托颌法

Post-reading

I. Check your Comprehension

Choose the best answer to complete each sentence with the information from the text.

1. Which is the first step of CPR?

   A. compressions   B. airway   C. breathing

2. If you see a person collapsed suddenly, what should you do first?

   A. Call someone for help.

   B. Check surroundings is or not safety.

   C. Immediate implementation of CPR.

3. The adult sternum should be depressed at least _____.

笔记

A. 2cm   B. 3～5cm   C. 5cm

4. If the person's neck is injured, what method is best to open the airway?

    A. jaw-thrust maneuver   B. head-tilt maneuver   C. chin-lift maneuver

5. What is called CPR's one operating cycle?

    A. 15 chests compressions followed by 2 rescue breaths.

    B. 2 rescue breaths followed by 15 chests compressions.

    C. 30 chests compressions followed by 2 rescue breaths.

II. Vocabulary Activities

Find a word or phrase from the box below to complete each sentence. Change word forms where necessary.

jaw	paramedic	emergency	resuscitation	compressions
palpate	sternum	perform	summarize	rescuer

1. An _____ is an unexpected and difficult or dangerous situation, especially an accident, which happens suddenly and which requires quick action to deal with it.

2. Always auscultate the abdomen before you _____ it.

3. The heart is posterior to the _____.

4. Basically, the article can be _____ four sentences.

5. If you _____ someone who has stopped breathing, you can sue mouth to mouth to do it.

6. She fell from a ladder, and broke her _____ bone.

7. After the earthquake in Wenchuan, there are many _____ to help.

8. An _____ said that he could have died if not been found so quickly.

9. If no pulse, initiate chest _____.

10. When you _____ a task or action, especially a complicated one, try you best to do it.

III. Supplementary

Text B

People who eat grains could get sick, and the doctor will give you some medication for your illness. Some drugs play a role in the treatment but also have adverse side effects. The following adverse reactions may occasionally occur: dryness of the mouth，thirst，drowsiness，fatigue，dizziness，heartburn，anorexia，abdominal discomfort and rash.

Pre-reading

1. What are common adverse drug reactions?

2. What are common routes of administration?

Medication Administration

Administering medication is the most commonly used method of treatment, including the treatment of diseases, reducing the symptoms, helping diagnose and maintain normal physiological function. In order that the medication is reasonable, safe and effective to the patient, you must know the medication condition of the patient as well as the pharmacology of the medication well.

ER-2-23
扫一扫 答案
"晓"

ER-2-24
扫一扫 练一
练

ER-2-25
扫一扫 听一
听

ER-2-26
扫一扫 知情
节

笔记

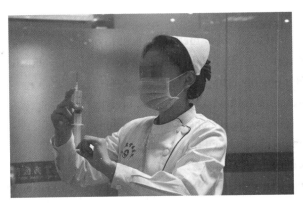

Fig. 2-4　parenteral injection

All medications have both desirable and undesirable effects. The desirable effect is commonly called therapeutic effect. Therapeutic effects of the drugs promote health, prevent disease, control disease processes. However, adverse effects sometimes occur that are usually undesirable and different from the therapeutic effect of the medication or any response to a medication which is noxious and unintended and occurs in doses for prevention, diagnosis, or treatment. The common adverse effects: side effects, toxic effects, allergic reaction, secondary reaction, drug dependency (physical and psychological).

There are many important principles for administering medications safely: Check medication orders before dispensing. If you find illegible, incomplete or otherwise questionable orders, you need to seek clarification before dispensing the medication. A physician determines the client's medication needs and orders medication. Usually, the order is written, although telephone and verbal orders are acceptable in a number of agencies. Nursing students need to know the agency policies about medication orders. Observe the "five rights" when administering the drug. Make sure to check three times: before administration, at the time of administration, and after administration. The "five rights" are right patient, right medication, right dose, right route, and right time.

A route of administration is the path by which a drug, poison, fluid, or other substance is taken into body. Routes of administration are classified into two categories: enteral and parenteral administration. Enteral administration refers to anything involving the stomach from the mouth to the rectum. There are three enteral routs of administration: Oral administration, Sublingual administration, and rectal administration. Parenteral administration is a method that drugs are injected into body fluids or tissues through a needle other than the digestive tract. Oral administration is a route that a drug is taken trough the mouth, it is a safe method and can reach different parts of the body via the bloodstream. Sublingual administration is a route that a drug diffuses into the blood through tissues under the tongue. You must tell the patient keep the drugs under the tongue and not swallow them. Rectal administration is a route that a drug absorbed by the rectum's blood vessels then flow into the body's circulation system.

(416 words)

Words in Focus

pharmacology /ˌfɑːməˈkɑːlədʒi/	n.	药理学；药物学
desirable /diˈzaiərəbəl/	adj.	可取的；令人满意的
therapeutic /ˌθɛrəˈpjutik/	adj.	治疗（学）的；疗法的

undesirable /ˌʌndiˈzaiərəbəl/	*adj.*	不良的；不合需要的
noxious /ˈnɔːkʃəs/	*adj.*	有害的；有毒的
unintended /ˌʌninˈtɛndid/	*adj.*	非故意的；无意识的
dose /doʊs/	*n.*	剂量，药量
dependency /diˈpendənsi/	*n.*	依赖
principle /ˈprinsipəl/	*n.*	原则，原理；准则，道义
dispense /diˈspɛns/	*v.*	分配；分给
prevention /priˈvɛnʃən/	*n.*	预防
illegible /iˈlɛdʒibəl/	*adj.*	无法辨认的
enteral /ˈentərəl/	*adj.*	肠的
parenteral /pæˈrentərəl/	*adj.*	肠外的
rectum /ˈrɛktəm/	*n.*	直肠

ER-2-27
扫一扫 读一读

ER-2-28
扫一扫 看一看

Useful Expressions

allergic reaction	变态反应
secondary reaction	继发反应
clarification from	澄清的
oral administration	口服给药
sublingual administration	舌下含化给药
rectal administration	直肠给药

Post-reading

I. Check your Comprehension

Read the following statements and then decide whether each of them is true or false based on the information from the text. Write T for true and F for false in the space provided.

_____ 1. Usually, the order is written, telephone and verbal orders are not acceptable.

_____ 2. All medications have both desirable and undesirable effects, you can change them.

_____ 3. If a drug through sublingual administration is given, it can be swallowed.

_____ 4. Sublingual administration is a route that a drug diffuses into the blood through tissues under the tongue.

_____ 5. If you find an illegible order, may be you need ask the doctor what it is.

II. Vocabulary activities

Find a word or phrase from the box below to complete each sentence. There are more words and phrases than you need to fill in all the sentences. Change word forms where is necessary.

prevent	therapeutic	diffuse	pharmacy	administration
precise	dependent	rectum	desirable	dispense

1. We worried about his _____ on his mother.

2. The doctor tells the patient to the _____ for her medicine.

3. Some shops gave wrong or inadequate advice when _____ homeopathic medicines.

4. The doctor told us that the drug has no _____ side-effects.

5. Lumbar disease morbidity is high and should take some measures to _____ and treatment in advance.

6. If patient's temperature can't be obtained by armpit, you can by _____ .

7. A drop of blood _____ in the water.

笔记

27

8. The preparation and _____ of medications are vital nursing functions.

9. The meeting began _____ at 5:00 p.m.

10. The nurse's training includes interpersonal communication skills,_____ interaction.

III. Supplementary

Part IV Writing

Breast Feeding Consultation

Instructions:

   A woman who has been pregnant for 30 weeks is confused with the problem of feeding the child in the future. She went to hospital for consultation. Please write about the contents of breast feeding in English, including three aspects:

1. *Feeding three forms: breast feeding, artificial feeding, mixed feeding.*

2. *The benefits of breast feeding.*

3. *What are artificial feeding and mixed feeding.*

_____

_____

_____

_____

_____

Part V Enriching your word power

director of the hospital	院长
director of administration	医务处主任
head of ...department	……科主任
specialist/expert	专家
doctor	医师
chief physician	主任医师
associate chief physician	副主任医师
attending doctor /doctor-in-charge	主治医师
resident doctor	住院医师
intern doctor	实习医师
physician	内科医师
surgeon	外科医师
gynecologist	妇科医师
obstetrician	产科医师
midwife	助产师
pediatrist	儿科医师
thoracic surgeon	胸外科医师
urological surgeon	泌尿外科医师

笔记

28

neurosurgeon	神经外科医师
plastic surgeon	矫形外科医师
anesthetist	麻醉科医师
e.n.t. doctor	耳鼻喉科医师
ophthalmologist	眼科医师
dentist	牙科医师
dermatologist	皮肤科医师
doctor for tuberculosis	结核科医师
gastroenterologist	消化科医师
doctor for infectious diseases	传染病科医师
dietician	营养科医师
orthopedist	骨科医师
radiologist	放射科医师
assistant doctor	医士
pharmacist	药剂师
assistant pharmacist	药剂士
laboratory technician	化验员
head of the nursing department	护理部主任
chief superintendent nurse /professor nurse	主任护师
head nurse	护士长
supervisor nurse /nurse-in-charge	主管护师
senior nurse /nurse practitioner	护师
registered nurse	注册护士
circulating nurse	巡回护师
student nurse	实习护士
assistant nurse	卫生员
professor of pharmacy	主任药师
pharmacist-in-charge	主管药师
pharmacist	药师
assistant pharmacist	药士
technologist	技师
technician	技士

Part Ⅵ　Exercise

Directions: *In this section, only one of the following options is correct, please choose.*

（纪敬敏　秦博文）

ER-2-32
扫一扫 看一看

29

Unit 3
Cardiology Department

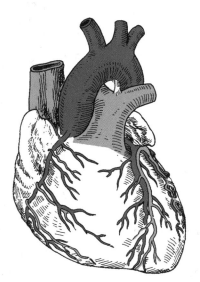

Fig. 3-1 our heart

A light heart lives long. 豁达者长寿。

——William Shakespeare（莎士比亚）

Learning Objectives

Skill focus

1. *Master the main symptoms of high blood pressure and myocardial infarction.*
2. *Know the basic nursing consultation related to myocarditis.*
3. *Learn some nursing interventions for the clients with heart failure.*

Language focus

1. *Describe the symptoms of high blood pressure and myocardial infarction with some medical terms.*
2. *Have ability of creating and guessing a new word using roots and prefix or suffix.*

Part Ⅰ Listening

This section is designed to test your ability to understand spoken English in nursing or medical contexts. You will hear a selection of recorded materials and you must answer the questions that accompany them. There are TWO parts in this section, Part A and Part B.

Part A

Words in Focus

weigh /weɪ/	v.	重量为······
dizzy /ˈdɪzi/	adj.	晕的
hypertension /ˌhaɪpə ˈtenʃn/	n.	高血压
peripheral /pəˈrɪfərəl/	adj.	外围的，外周的
metabolic /ˌmetəˈbɒlɪk/	adj.	新陈代谢的；变化的

Useful Expressions

blood pressure	血压
have risk of	有······的危险

Text

Directions: *In this section you will hear a short passage, at the end of the passage, one or more questions will be asked about what was said, decide which the best answer is.*

Background:

Mr. Smith is not very well these days, he often feels tired and dizzy. Now he is consulting with the Dr.

Comprehension of the Text

1. Where does the conversation probably take place?

   A. at Mr. Smith home　　　　B. in outpatient clinic　　　C. in the operation room

2. What is the blood pressure level for a doctor begins to concern?

   A. It's consistently more than 180/110mmHg.

   B. It is around 120/80mmHg.

   C. It is greater than 140/90mmHg.

3. What may cause hypertension mentioned in the dialogue?

   A. overwork　　　　　　　B. too much exercise　　　　C. sleep quality

4. Overweight may increase _____ and _____ changes.

   A. peripheral resistance, body circulation

   B. the risk of heart attack, metabolic

   C. peripheral resistance, metabolic

5. Which measure is not mentioned to help patients with hypertension?

   A. to go to bed early　　　B. to do more exercises　　　C. to decrease butter intake

Part B

Words in Focus

electrocardiogram /iˌlektroʊˈkɑːdiəgræm/	n.	心电图
voltage /ˈvəʊltɪdʒ; ˈvɒltɪdʒ/	n.	电位
depolarization /diːˈpoʊləraɪˈzeɪʃən/	n.	去极化
repolarization /riːˌpoʊləraɪˈzeɪʃən/	n.	复极化
complex /kɒmˈpleks/	n.	群；复合体
atria /ˈeɪtriə/	n.	心房（atrium 的复数）
systole /ˈsɪstəli/	n.	收缩
ventricular /venˈtrɪkjələ/	adj.	心室的

ER-3-1
扫一扫 读一读

ER-3-2
扫一扫 看一看

ER-3-3
扫一扫 听一听

ER-3-4
扫一扫 知情节

ER-3-5
扫一扫 读一读

ER-3-6
扫一扫 看一看

笔记

impulse /ˈimˌpʌls/	n.	冲动，搏动
segment /ˈsɛgmənt/	n.	分段
clinically /ˈklinikli/	adv.	临床地
congenital /kənˈdʒɛnitl/	adj.	先天的

Useful Expressions

corresponds to	对应
conduction system	传导系统
electrolyte imbalance	电解质失衡

Text

ER-3-7
扫一扫 听一听

ER-3-8
扫一扫 知情节

Directions: *In this section you will hear a short passage, at the end of the passage, you are asked to complete the missing parts accordingly. You will hear the passage twice.*

Background:

You are attending a training session, the following is a brief introduction of electrocardiogram.

Comprehension of the Text

The Electrocardiogram

An electrocardiogram (ECG) is the visual representation of the heart's conduction system，which measures and monitors the (1)_____ of the heart through the skin. The ECG produces a (2) _____ in response to the electrical changes taking place within the heart.

The first part of the wave, called the P wave, is (3) _____ that corresponds to the depolarization of the atria during atrial systole. P-R interval represents (4) _____ through the conduction system; The next part of the ECG wave is the QRS complex which features a small drop in voltage (Q)，a large voltage peak (R) and another small drop in voltage (S). The QRS complex represents ventricular depolarization during ventricular systole. The atria also repolarize (5) _____, but have almost no effect on the ECG because they are (6) _____ than the ventricles. The final part of the EKG wave is the T wave, a small peak that follows the QRS complex. T wave represents (7) _____. S-T segment represents early ventricle repolarization.

(8) _____ between the waves of the ECG can be used clinically to diagnose the effects of heart attacks, congenital heart problems, and electrolyte imbalances.

Part II Speaking

This section is designed to test your speaking ability. After learning the following conversation A and B you will have the ability of speaking skill in medical and nursing working and try to do the following speaking tasks.

Conversation 1

Myocardial Infarction

Mr. Morgan *and his friend are walking along the Connecticut Ave, and of sudden, he has passed out on the street. He seems painful and abnormally uncomfortable awareness of breathing. He is breaking into a cold sweat with lips cyanosis. He pressed his chest and can't speak out a word. He is soon sent to the hospital and has taken the first aid. After a while, he is awake.*

笔记

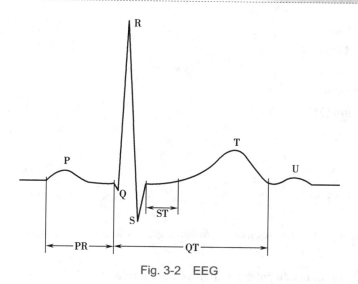

Fig. 3-2 EEG

Doctor:	Hello, Mr. Morgan. How are you feeling now?
Mr. Morgan:	A little better.
Doctor:	Has the chest pain relieved a little?
Mr. Morgan:	Yes, it has. What's wrong with me?
Doctor:	I think it might be something serious just now. You've just had a myocardial infarction.
Mr. Morgan:	Myocardial infarction! Oh，my God.
Doctor:	Yes, that's right. Have you ever had any heart attack before?
Mr. Morgan:	None. But I am not feeling well these couple of days.
Doctor:	Have you noticed any symptoms recently?
Mr. Morgan:	Well, I had been having chest pains on and off for the past week or so. It lasts for 2-3 minutes at a time and I usually get pretty sweaty, nauseous, and even have trouble breathing. It seems to come on when I'm doing something, like walking upstairs, but it goes away as soon as I sit down.
Doctor:	En, I see, they are all typical signs and symptoms of cardiovascular assessment. Does anyone in your family suffer from heart disease with things like high blood pressure, heart attacks, arrhythmia, heart failure, high cholesterol, or the like?
Mr. Morgan:	My father suffered from myocardial infarction and I think his heart disease eventually failed him, which is probably where I got it from.
Doctor:	Maybe it is.
Mr. Morgan:	What should I do next，doctor?
Doctor:	We will do more examination to make further diagnosis. You should stay in bed for at least one week and don't do much exertion. Please be low in cholesterol and sodium. If you feel any uncomfortable, please let me and the nurse know.
Mr. Morgan:	Yes, I will. Thank you, doctor.

(308 words)

Words in Focus

relieve /ri'liv/	v.	缓解，解除
nauseous /'nɔːsjəs/	adj.	感到恶心的

笔记

33

ER-3-11
扫一扫 读一读

ER-3-12
扫一扫 看一看

arrhythmia /əˈriθmiə/	n.	心律失常
cholesterol /kəˈlestərɔːl/	n.	胆固醇
sodium /ˈsoʊdiəm/	n.	钠

Useful Expressions

myocardial infarction (MI)	心肌梗死
short of breath	气短
chest pain	胸痛
on and off	断断续续
cardiovascular assessment	心血管疾病评估

I. Free talk

Directions: *Work in pairs and discuss the following questions after learning to the recording of* Dialogue One.

1. What are the symptoms of a patient with myocardial infarction?

_____

_____

2. How to give the first aid for a myocardial infarction patient?

_____

_____

3. Is there any requirement for myocardial infarction patients' daily diet?

_____

_____

II. Comprehension of the Text

Directions: *Choose the best answer according to the conversation.*

1. Why was Mr. Morgan sent to the hospital?
    A. He has a chest pain.
    B. He has a heart attack.
    C. He feels light-head for overwork.

2. Is there anyone suffer from heart disease in Mr. Morgan's family？
    A. Yes, there is one person mentioned.
    B. No, one person is mentioned but he has no relation to heart attack.
    C. No, no one is mentioned at all.

3. Which symptom is not mentioned by Mr. Morgan?
    A. chest pain for a week
    B. short of breath
    C. vomit and feel sick

4. What is the suggestion of the doctor?
    A. Do exercises as possible as he can.
    B. Stay in bed for a least one week.
    C. Eat with low cholesterol and sodium in diet.

5. When may this dialogue take place?
    A. before hospitalization
    B. before being discharged from hospital
    C. during the treatment

ER-3-13
扫一扫 答案
"晓"

笔记

Conversation 2

Myocarditis

ER-3-14
扫一扫 听一
听

ER-3-15
扫一扫 知情
节

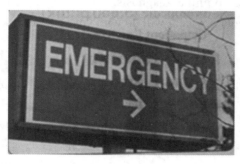

Fig. 3-3   emergency

Wang Zheng, 28 years old, is a Chinese oversea student in America. One month ago he had a bad cold with high fever, cough, vomiting and diarrhea. *With the help of his friends, he feels much better from illness. Unfortunately, he* began to feel palpitation and short of breath the other days. *He made an appointment with the doctor beforehand and now he is in the doctor's office.*

Wang Zheng: Doctor, I'm not feeling well today.

Doctor: Can you tell me what the problem is?

Wang Zheng: Yes, I had a high fever, cough, vomiting and diarrhea, etc. I've thought I had a bad cold.

Doctor: When did this happen?

Wang Zheng: It started from last month. At the beginning I had a sore throat.

Doctor: Yes, let me see. Open your mouth and say "Ah".

Wang Zheng： "Ah..."

Doctor: It seems a little red.

Wang Zheng: Yes, much better now. But more uncomfortable about my heart.

Doctor: Your heart? Any symptoms?

Wang Zheng: I begin to feel palpitation and short of breath recently. Sometimes I even cough up at night. My chest pains aggravating when taking a deep breath and rolling-off.

Doctor: There may be a little trouble with your heart. You have to take an echocardiography examination, which is a necessary diagnostic test.

Wang Zheng: Thank you.

After a while...

Doctor: The result of your electrocardiogram indicates that your ST segment depression and T-wave lowering.

Wang Zheng: It seems too complex. What's wrong with me?

Doctor: It seems like a myocarditis.

Wang Zheng: Oh, I am scared.

Doctor: I understand you, but don't be afraid, take it easy. Myocarditis (esp Viral myocarditis) is a common disease, especially in the winter and spring seasons with the early symptom of the upper respiratory tract infection and intestinal infection, and then cause arrhythmia in the way of palpitation.

笔记

Wang Zheng: Well ... what should I do next?

Doctor: You have to stay in bed and get a good rest at least for 3weeks. Meanwhile decrease physical exertion before your heart recovered. Tomorrow we will do a laboratory test to further diagnosis.

Wang Zheng: Thanks for your advice. I will do with your guidance.

(309 words)

Words in Focus

myocarditis /ˌmaiouka:ˈdaitis/	*n.*	心肌炎
vomit /ˈvɑ:mit/	*v.*	使呕吐；吐出
diarrhea /ˌdaiəˈriə/	*n.*	腹泻；痢疾
palpitation /ˌpælpiˈteiʃən/	*n.*	心悸
aggravate /ˈæɡrəveit/	*v.*	加剧；恶化

Useful Expressions

roll-off	翻身
respiratory tract infection	上呼吸道感染
intestinal infection	肠道感染

I. Free talk

Directions: *Work in pairs and discuss the following questions after learning.*

1. What are the main symptoms of Wang Zheng?

_____

2. What kind of examinations will be taken for Mr. Zhang according to the doctor's advice?

_____

3. What should a myocarditis patient pay attention to in daily life?

_____

II. Comprehension of the Text

Directions: *According to the conversation and complete the table.*

NAME		SEX	
AGE		OCCUPATION	
COMPLAINT	1. 2. 3.		
EXAMINATION	1. 2. 3.		
DIAGNOSIS	1. 2.		
ADVICE	1. 2.		

ER-3-16
扫一扫 读一读

ER-3-17
扫一扫 看一看

ER-3-18
扫一扫 答案 "晓"

笔记

Part Ⅲ   Reading

Text A

ER-3-19
扫一扫 听一
听

ER-3-20
扫一扫 知情
节

> Our heart sits in the middle of our chest and pumps blood. It never stops, and over our lifetime it will pump 175 million liters of blood. Imagine the amount of water that falls over Niagara falls in a few minutes. Remarkable! Now we will learn more about the heart anatomy and how the heart works.
>
> ***Pre-reading***
>
> 1. Do you know the basic anatomical structure of your heart?
> 2. Do you know systemic circulation and pulmonary circulation?
> 3. How to understand the saying A light heart lives long.

Our Heart

No organ quite symbolizes love like the heart. One reason may be that our heart helps us live, by moving 5 liters of blood through almost 100,000 kilometers of blood vessels every single minute! It has to do this all day, every day, without ever taking a vacation! Now that is true love.

Our heart is a muscular organ about the size of a closed fist that functions as the body's circulatory pump. It is located in the middle of the mediastinum, where the lungs partially overlap it. On its superior end, the base of the heart is attached to the aorta, pulmonary arteries and veins, and the vena cava. The inferior tip of the heart, known as the apex, rests just superior to the diaphragm.

Basically, our heart is divided into four chambers. The two upper chambers, called atria, are joined to the two lower chambers, called ventricles. An internal partition separates the left atrium and ventricle from the right atrium and ventricle.

The blood comes back to the right atrium and is pumped through the tricuspid valve into the right ventricle. The atria receive blood that is returning to the heart, which then flows into the ventricles-the heart's pumps. The right and left ventricles are larger than the right and left atria because they are responsible for the pumping action of the heart. The right ventricle pumps de-oxygenated blood away from the heart through the T-shaped pulmonary artery. By the time blood arrives in the lungs the body has taken out most of oxygen and made use of it for tissue function. In a healthy heart, the blood flows efficiently through the heart to the lungs, which re-oxygenate the blood and return it to the heart through the pulmonary vein. This is a relative short route, we call it pulmonary circulation.

Oxygenated blood enters the heart through the left atrium and is pumped to the left ventricle. The left ventricle is encased in thicker cardiac muscle than the right side because it has to pump oxygenated blood around the entire body via the aorta, the largest artery of the body. After whole body traveling, the poor-oxygenated blood comes back to the right atrium, which is known as systemic circulation. The cardiac cycle relies on the efficiency of the four

笔记

valves between the atria, the ventricles and the pulmonary blood vessels. These valves open to the left in sufficient blood flow to fill each heart chamber and then shut to prevent the backflow of blood. Irregularities in blood flow because of blockages in the blood vessels can lead to heart disease.

(431 words)

Words in Focus

ER-3-21
扫一扫 读一
读

symbolize /'simbəlaiz/	v.	象征
circulatory /'sə:kjələtɔri/	adj.	循环的
mediastinum /ˌmi:diæs'tainəm/	n.	纵隔
overlap /ˌouvə'læp/	v.	重叠，相交
apex /'eipɛks/	n.	心尖
diaphragm /'daiəˌfræm/	n.	横膈膜
oxygenated /'ɒksidʒəneitid/	adj.	含氧的
vein /vein/	n.	静脉
artery /'ɑ:təri/	n.	动脉
aorta /ei'ɔ:tə/	n.	主动脉
backflow /'bæk'flou/	n.	回流
blockage /'blɑ:kidʒ/	n.	堵塞物，阻塞

ER-3-22
扫一扫 看一
看

Useful Expressions

muscular organ	肌肉器官
be attached to	与……相连
vena cava	腔静脉
tricuspid valve	三尖瓣
pulmonary artery	肺动脉

Post-reading

I. Comprehension of the text

Ⅰ) **Choose the best answer to complete each sentence with the information from the text.**

1. Why does our heart stand for love?

    A. Because it looks like heart-shaped.

    B. Because our heart transports blood every day without any rest.

    C. Because we love our heart better than any other organ.

2. Which statement is not true according to paragraph 2?

    A. Our heart is a muscular organ about the size of a closed fist.

    B. The heart is located in the middle of the mediastinum and the lungs.

    C. Pulmonary arteries connect with the base of the heart, diaphragm is attached to the apex.

3. How does blood travel in a pulmonary circulation?

    A. right atrium-right ventricle-pulmonary artery-tissue function-pulmonary vein-left atrium

    B. left ventricle-aorta-tissue function-vena cava-right atrium

    C. right ventricle-right atrium-pulmonary artery-tissue function-aorta-left atrium

4. Which Statement is not right about left ventricle?

    A. The left ventricle is larger than the left atrium.

    B. The left ventricle pumps oxygenated blood around the entire body via the aorta.

    C. The left ventricular pumps de-oxygenated blood away from the heart through the T-shaped pulmonary artery.

5. What is the type of this passage?

    A. popular science   B. practical writing   C. science fiction

Ⅱ) Read the following statements and then decide whether each of them is true or false based on the information from the text. Write T for true and F for false in the space provided.

_____1. The base of the heart connects with the aorta, pulmonary arteries and veins, the inferior tip of the heart rests on the top of the diaphragm.

_____2. The two upper chambers are atria, the two lower chambers are ventricles.

_____3. The blood enters to the right atrium and is pumped into the right ventricle through the mitral valve.

_____4. The right ventricle pumps oxygenated blood to the heart through the T-shaped pulmonary artery.

_____5. The cardiac cycle relies on the efficiency of the four valves between the atria, the ventricles and the pulmonary blood vessels.

II. Vocabulary activities

Find a word or phrase from the box below to complete each sentence. There are more words and phrases than you need to fill in all the sentences. Change word forms where necessary.

symbolize	overlap	diaphragm	oxygenate	muscular organ
circulatory	aorta	ventricle	blockage	blood vessels

1. The crane _____ good fortune, peace and longevity.

2. The heart rate and general movement in the _____ system slows due to the decreased demand for blood while sitting.

3. The needs of patients invariably _____.

4. The treatment is used to _____ the blood of patients when the lungs or heart stop working normally.

5. When we inhale, our lungs fill with air, which press the _____ downward.

6. The right _____ pump sends blood out of the heart to the lungs.

7. The logical treatment is to remove this _____.

8. The heart is a _____ that contracts rhythmically.

9. Caffeine dilates _____, thus increasing the flow of blood and oxygen to muscles.

10. These medications reduce the strength and frequency of heartbeats, reducing stress on the wall of the _____.

ER-3-23
扫一扫 答案
"晓"

ER-3-24
扫一扫 练一
练

III. Supplementary

Text B

Heart failure is a condition in which the heart is unable to pump blood efficiently, meaning that it cannot meet the body's demands for blood and oxygen. It has attacked more than 8 million people around China by the end of 2014, which is twice as much as the number in 2003. The indicators of risk are sounding the alarm.

笔记

ER-3-25
扫一扫 听一
听

ER-3-26
扫一扫 知情
节

Pre-reading

1. Do you know the type of heart failure?

2. Do you know the early symptoms of heart failure?

Heart Failure

Heart failure (HF), often referred to as congestive heart failure (CHF), occurs when the heart is unable to pump sufficiently to maintain blood flow to meet the body's needs. It is a common and potentially fatal condition. In developed countries, around 2% of adults have heart failure and in those over the age of 65, this increases to 6%～10%. It has attacked more than 8 million people around China by the end of 2014 which is similar to the risks with a number of types of cancer.

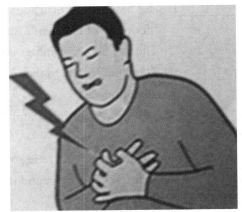

Fig. 3-4   heart failure

Signs and symptoms of heart failure commonly include shortness of breath, excessive tiredness, and leg swelling. The shortness of breath is usually worse with exercise, while lying down, it may wake the person up at night. A limited ability to exercise is also a common feature.

According to its symptom and physique, it can be divided into left heart failure, right heart failure and whole heart failure. Left-sided heart failure occurs when there is a weakness in the left ventricle, which cannot adequately pump blood returning from the lungs into the arterial circulation. This blood backs up into the lung tissue and leads to pulmonary edema. Right-sided heart failure is due to the weakness in the right ventricle and subsequent inability to circulate the systematic circulation and results in dependent edema. A whole heart failure patient is often suffered from both left heart failure and right heart failure.

The causes of heart failure are divided into primary causes and precipitating causes. The primary causes of heart failure include conditions that overload the heart, affect the cardiac rhythm or conduction or decrease the ability of the heart to contract. These include coronary artery disease, rheumatic heart disease, arrhythmias, myocarditis, hypertension and structural heart defects. The precipitating causes of heart failure include hypertension and hypothyroidism, obesity, anemia, pregnancy and environmental and emotional stress.

The condition is diagnosed based on the history of the symptoms and a physical examination by echocardiography. Blood tests, electrocardiography, and chest radiography may be useful to determine the underlying cause. Treatment depends on the severity and cause of the disease. In people with chronic stable mild heart failure, treatment commonly consists of lifestyle modifications such as stopping smoking, physical exercise, and dietary changes, as well as medications. In those with heart failure due to left ventricular dysfunction, angiotensin along with beta blockers are recommended.

For nursing a heart failure patient, a nurse should do some interventions. Firstly the nurse should actively work to improve existing alternations in cardiac output by reducing cardiac workload, promoting venous return and minimizing myocardial oxygen requirements. Secondly, the patient may be more comfortable and better able to rest while receiving oxygen. Oxygen

笔记

is usually administered by nasal cannula at 2 to 6L/min. Thirdly, to decrease excessive fluid volumes. Nurses work with the patient to determine how to best manage fluid and sodium restrictions. Lastly, the nurse should explain the importance of moderate exercise to patient which may help prevent patient from being afraid to perform daily activities. Cardiac rehabilitation programs are especially beneficial for patients who are anxious about exercising on their own.

(494 words)

Words in Focus

congestive /kən'dʒestiv/	*adj.*	充血的，充血性的
swelling /'swɛliŋ/	*n.*	膨大，肿胀
adequately /ˌ'ædikwitli/	*adv.*	适当地，充分地
precipitating /pri'sipiteitiŋ/	*adj.*	促成的，诱因的
rheumatic /ru'mætik/	*adj.*	风湿病的
hypothyroidism /ˌhaipou'θairɔidizəm/	*n.*	甲状腺功能减退
obesity /o'bisəti/	*n.*	肥胖症，肥胖
anemia /ə'ni:miə/	*n.*	贫血
angiotensin /ˌændʒiou'tensən/	*n.*	血管紧张素
intervention /ˌintə'venʃn/	*n.*	干预，介入
moderate /'mɔ:dərət/	*adj.*	中等的；有节制的
restriction /ri'strikʃən/	*n.*	限制，束缚

ER-3-27
扫一扫 读一读

ER-3-28
扫一扫 看一看

Useful Expressions

pulmonary edema	肺水肿
rheumatic heart disease	风湿性心脏病
chronic dysfunction	慢性功能障碍
cardiac rehabilitation	心脏康复

Post-reading

I. Comprehension of the text

Choose the best answer to complete each sentence with the information from the text.

1. Heart failure _____.

    A. is a common and potentially fatal condition

    B. has attacked nearly 8 million people around China by the end of 2014

    C. has attacked around 2% of adults over the age of 65 in developing countries

2. Which symptom of heart failure is not mentioned in this passage?

    A. excessive tiredness and leg swelling

    B. diarrhea

    C. a limited ability to exercise

3. What statement is true about left heart failure?

    A. It occurs when the left ventricle cannot pump blood returning from the lungs into the arterial circulation.

    B. When it occurs, the blood backs up into the body tissue and leads to dependent edema.

    C. It is due to the weakness in the right ventricle and subsequent inability to circulate the systematic circulation and results in pulmonary edema.

4. What is the principle of treatment about heart failure?

    A. People with heart failure due to left ventricular dysfunction, should make lifestyle

笔记

modifications and dietary changes.

  B. People with chronic stable mild heart failure, angiotensin along with beta blockers are recommended.

  C. Treatment of heart failure depends on the severity and cause of the disease.

5. How should the nurse do to care for a heart failure patient according to this passage?

  A. Mask oxygen inhalation is administered at 2 to 6L/min.

  B. The nurse should improve existing alternations in cardiac output.

  C. The nurse should try to increase fluid volumes.

II. Check your vocabulary

Find a word or phrase from the box below to complete each sentence. There are more words and phrases than you need to fill in all the sentences. Change word forms where necessary.

| congestive | intervention | chronic | restrictions | moderate |
| dietary | dysfunction | obesity | swelling | pulmonary edema |

1. According to published reports, Felt died of _____ heart failure.

2. Let me know how you try to simplify your _____ needs approach.

3. Teenagers who mistakenly perceive themselves as overweight are actually at greater risk of _____ as adults, new research has revealed.

4. This blocks the flow of blood to the brain and other organs, and causes anaemia, respiratory problems and brain _____.

5. They think his illness is acute rather than _____.

6. Do you have age _____?

7. The lungs should be examined for possible _____.

8. The _____ affected the entire leg.

9. It's very clear that you don't need any advice. What you need is _____.

10. Formal physical therapy may _____ to your treatment.

III. Supplementary

Part IV   Writing

Writing an Admission Record

Instructions:

  An admission record or in-patient is a part of medical record which is used somewhat to describe the systematic documentation of a single patient's medical history and care procedures when he or she is admitted. The admission record includes a variety of types of "notes": symptoms, inquiry, charts and images etc, so as to identify the patient, to support the diagnosis, and to justify the treatment. But for a brief admission record, the patient's basic information, chief complaint, signs and symptoms, diagnosis and nursing instruction are all necessary points.

  Admission records have traditionally been compiled and maintained by health care providers, but advances in online data storage have led to the development of personal health records (PHR) that are maintained by patients themselves, often on third-party websites.

  Because many consider the information in the records to be sensitive personal information,

ER-3-29
扫一扫 答案
"晓"

ER-3-30
扫一扫 练一
练

笔记

so the admission records are demanded to keep well without leaking of privacy.

Sentence Patterns

1. No history of ... 无……史。

   No history of infective diseases. 无感染史。

   No allergy history of food and drugs. 无食物、药物过敏史。

2. well +V. ed 良好的……

   He is well developed and moderately nourished.

   他身体健康，营养适度。

   It's worth making an effort to look well-dressed.

   在衣着打扮上花些功夫是值得的。

Examples:

Patient　Admission Record	
Patient: John Davis	**Age:** Eighty
Gender: Male	**Date of Admission:** July10,2015
Chief Complaint: 1). Upper bellyache ten days; 2). Haematemesis, hemafecia and unconsciousness for four hours.	
Signs and symptoms: 1).Upper bellyache for ten days. He didn't pay attention; 2). Faint and reject lots of blood and gore at 6:00 this morning; 3). Begin to have hemafecia; 4). Does not urinate since the disease coming on.	
Diagnosis: 1). Upper gastrointestine hemorrhage; 2). Exsanguine shock.	
Nursing instruction: 1). Lying in horizontal position without pillow ; 2). Clearance the respiratory tract and uptake oxygen; 3). Diuretic drugs and cardiac drugs are recommended; 4). Observe vital signs; 5). Liquid diet may be appropriate when there is minimal hemorrhage.	

Practice

Mr.Brown, age 56, an engineer, complains that he has had brief episodes of chest pain since his admission on Otc.20, 2015. He realizes that he has a heart attack. He spent 2 days in the coronary care unit (CCU) and then moved to a step-down unit.

Mr. Brown's general health has been excellent, with no major health problems. He says that I have never been sick a day in my life, except for colds. Mr. Brown follows no special diet; enjoys his wife's cooking; began reducing the amount of cholesterol in his diet about 3 years ago. Recently, his appetite has been only fair, "I'm eating, but not enjoying my food". Usually sleeps 6～7 hours at night. He has no trouble falling asleep. But at present, he has been requesting a more sleeping pill at night, not able to sleep well with one pillow.

Mr. Brown has three nursing diagnoses:

1. Pain related to inadequate blood flow to myocardial tissue. And possible interventions will be

   A. Obtain ECG.

   B. Administer oxygen as ordered.

   C. Administer nitroglycerin as ordered.

   D. Relieve anxiety and offer reassurance.

2. Activity Intolerance related to imbalance between oxygen supply and demand. The possible interventions include:

　　A. Assess level of tolerance to specific activities and monitor heart rate and blood pressure before, during and after activity.

　　B. Prescribe a progressive activity and exercise program for each phase of recovery.

　　C. Instruct the patient about energy conservation and rest requirements.

3. Knowledge Deficit related to lack of information about myocardial infarction, treatment regimen, risk factor modification and cardiac rehabilitation. The nurse should develop a teaching plan including:

　　A. normal anatomy, physiology of the heart, and myocardial infarction

　　B. methods used for risk factor modification such as stop-smoking program, diet modification, weight control, stress reduction and activity/exercise program

Summarize a brief medical record according to the above passage

Patient Admission Record			
Patient		**Age**	
Gender		**Occupation**	
Date of Admission			
Chief Complaint			
Signs and symptoms			
Past history			
Diagnosis			
Nursing interventions			

ER-3-31
扫一扫 答案
"晓"

Part Ⅴ　Enriching your word power

1.	cardi(o)-		心脏，心
	cardiocinetic /kɑːdiːəʊkaiˈnetik/ 同 cardiokinetic		强心药
	cardiomyopathy /ˌkɑːdiəʊmaiˈɒpəθi/		心肌病
2.	atri(o)-		心房
	atriomegaly /ˈeitriəmegəli/		心房肥大
	sinoatrial /sainəʊˈetriəl/		窦房的
3.	ventricul(o)-		室（脑室，心室）
	ventriculopuncture /venˈtrikjuləʊpʌnktʃə/		脑室穿刺术
	ventriculotomy /ventrikjuˈləʊtəʊmi/		心室切开术；脑室切开术
4.	arteri(o)-		动脉
	arteriosclerosis /ɑːˌtiəriəʊskləˈrəʊsis/		动脉硬化

笔记

arteriogram /ɑːˈtiəriəugræm/	动脉脉搏图
5. ven(o)-; phleb(o)-	静脉
venostasis /viːnəˈsteisis/	静脉郁滞
phlebitis /fləˈbaitis/	静脉炎
6. sten(o)-	狭窄，狭小
stenosis /stiˈnəusis/	（器官）狭窄
stenocardia /stenəˈkɑːdiə/ 同 angina pectoris	心绞痛
7. brady-	慢
bradycardia /brædiˈkɑːdiə/	心动过缓，心搏徐缓
bradyesthesia /breidiesˈθiːziə/	感觉过慢，感觉迟钝
8. tachy-	快，快速
tachycardia /ˌtækiˈkɑːdiə/	心动过速
tachypnea /tækipˈniːə/	呼吸促迫，呼吸急促
9. olig(o)-	少，缺少
oligoamnios /ɒliˈgəumniːəuz/	羊水过少
oliguria /ɒliˈgjuəriə/	尿过少，少尿（症）
10. angi (o); vas(o); vascul(o)-	血管
angiogram /ˈændʒiə(u)græm/	血管造影
vasodilator /ˌveizəudaiˈleitə/	血管扩张药
vasculopathy /ˈvæskjuləupəθi/	血管病
11. aort(o)-	主动脉
aortitis /ˌeiɔːˈtaitis/	主动脉炎
aortosclerosis /eiɔːtəuskləˈrəusis/	主动脉硬化
12. sphygm(o)-	脉搏
sphygmogram /ˈsfigməgræm/	脉搏描记曲线
sphygmology /ˌsfigˈmɒlədʒi/	脉学，脉搏学

Part Ⅵ Exercise

Directions: *In this section, only one of the following options is correct, please choose.*

（保　静　吕小君）

ER-3-32
扫一扫 看一
看

笔记

Unit 4
Respiratory Department

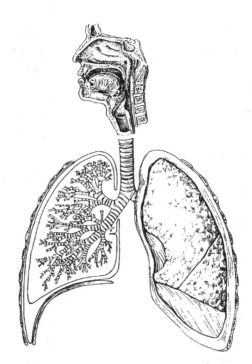

Fig. 4-1   respiratory department

Cheerfulness is the promoter of health. 心情愉快是健康的增进剂。

——Joseph Addison（约瑟夫·阿狄生）

Learning Objectives

Skill focus

1. *Understanding the structure and function of the respiratory system.*
2. *Mastering the steps of the cultivation of the sputum and related matters.*

Language focus

1. *Describe one of the medical terms you have learnt in this unit.*
2. *Have ability of creating and guessing a new word using roots and prefix or suffix.*

Part I   Listening

This section is designed to test your ability to understand spoken English in nursing or medical contexts. You will hear a selection of recorded materials and you must answer the

questions that accompany them. There are TWO parts in this section, Part A and Part B.

Part A

Words in Focus

bacteria /bæk'tiəriə/	*n.*	细菌
sampling /'sæmpliŋ/	*n.*	抽样，取样
pneumonia /njuːˈməʊniə/	*n.*	肺炎；急性肺炎
expectorate /ikˈspɛktəreit/	*v.*	咳出，吐痰
thick /θik/	*adj.*	稠密的；不透明的
sensitivity /'sɛnsi'tiviti/	*n.*	灵敏性；感光度
cabinet /'kæbinit/	*n.*	内阁；柜橱
pathogenic /ˌpæθəˈdʒɛnik/	*adj.*	引起疾病的
transmit /trænz'mit/	*v.*	传播，发射；传递，传染
pathogens /'pæθədʒəns/	*n.*	病菌，病原体

Useful Expressions

for this reason	以此，为此
biochemical test	生化检验
antimicrobial agent	抗菌剂
respiratory flora	呼吸道菌群

Text

Directions: *In this section you will hear a short passage, at the end of the passage, one or more questions will be asked about what was said, decide which the best answer is.*

Comprehension of the text

1. Sputum is a _____ produced in the lungs and in the adjacent airways.

   A. solid   B. thick fluid   C. transparent liquid

2. In a hospital setting, a sputum culture is most commonly ordered if a patient has a _____.

   A. cancer   B. appendicitis   C. pneumonia

3. The Infectious Diseases Society of America recommends that sputum cultures be done in pneumonia requiring hospitalization, while the American College of Chest Physicians does not.

   A. Yes   B. No   C. Not mentioned

4. Laboratory processing of sputum for respiratory pathogens is performed with the aid of a _____ safety cabinet.

   A. biological   B. chemical   C. physical

5. A sample of sputum is placed in a _____ container and sent to the laboratory for testing.

   A. dark   B. warm   C. sterile

Part B

Words in Focus

feverish /'fivəriʃ/	*adj.*	发热的；极度兴奋的
phlegm /flɛm/	*n.*	痰；黏液

ER-4-3
扫一扫 听一听

ER-4-4
扫一扫 知情节

ER-4-5
扫一扫 读一读

ER-4-6
扫一扫 看一看

笔记

| whitish /'waitiʃ/ | adj. | 带白色的；发白的 |
| rimifon /'rimifən/ | n. | 异烟肼 |

Useful Expressions

injection of streptomycin   注射链霉素

Text

Directions: *In this section you will hear a short passage, at the end of the passage, one or more questions will be asked about what was said, decide which the best answer is.*

Background:

    The following conversation is about lung test. Listen to it carefully and choose the right answer to each question.

Comprehension of the text

1. Which of the following is not one of the symptoms of patient with tuberculosis?

    A. feeling weak   B. cough   C. emesis

2. Which method can judge whether patient is suffering from tuberculosis?

    A. urinalysis   B. X-ray   C. B ultrasonic

3. Which of the following is the symptom of patient with tuberculosis?

    A. blood-stained sputum   B. headache   C. toothache

4. If the patient is suffering from severe tuberculosis, how much time is needed to treat the patient?

    A. about six months   B. about one year   C. about two weeks

5. Which of the following drugs can be used to treat tuberculosis?

    A. insulin   B. aspirin   C. rimifon and streptomycin

Part Ⅱ   Speaking

    This section is designed to test your speaking ability. After learning the following conversation A and B you will have the ability of speaking skill in medical and nursing working and try to do the following speaking tasks.

Conversation 1

Treatment of Patients with Bronchitis and Pneumonia

    A patient goes to the hospital. The doctor tells him that he has been infected with pneumonia and how he will be treated.

Patient: I can't stop coughing, doctor.

Doctor: When did the cough begin?

Patient: It started a week ago, but it has been getting worse since yesterday.

Doctor: Do you cough up any phlegm?

Patient: Yes.

Doctor: What color is it?

Patient: Yellow.

Doctor: Do you have a fever?

Patient:　Yes, I feel feverish.

Doctor:　Have you felt shivery?

Patient:　Yes, sometimes.

Doctor:　Do you smoke?

Patient:　Yes, I do. I'm a heavy smoker.

Doctor:　Let me examine you. Lie down on the bed please. Take your shoes off and unbutton your shirt, please.

Doctor:　Your heart seems to be normal. Your breathing is low. I can hear moist rales over the left lung base. I'll take a white blood count and give you a fluoroscopic examination immediately.

Doctor:　Here are the slips for blood text and fluoroscopic examination. First, please go to the cashier to pay the fee, then go to the laboratory for blood test and X-ray room for the fluoroscopic examination. I'll wait here for the reports.

Patient:　Here are the reports, is there anything wrong?

Doctor:　I am sure it's pneumonia. Don't be alarmed, but you should be admitted to hospital and treated with penicillin and streptomycin. For the time being you should stop smoking. After several days you'll feel much better.

(254 words)

Words in Focus

shivery /ˈʃivəri/	adj.	颤抖的；发抖的
rale /ˈrɑːl/	n.	啰音；水泡音，肺的诊音
fluoroscopic /flu(:)ərəˈskɒpik/	adj.	荧光镜的；荧光检查法的
streptomycin /ˈstreptəˈmaisin/	n.	链霉素
Penicillin /ˈpɛniˈsilin/	n.	青霉素；盘尼西林

Useful Expressions

| lie down | 躺下 |
| be admitted to | 住进 |

ER-4-11
扫一扫 读一读

ER-4-12 ·
扫一扫 看一看

I. Free talk

Directions: Work in pairs and discuss the following questions after learning to the recording of Dialogue One.

1. According to the article, please describe the symptoms of pneumonia.

_____

_____

_____

2. According to the article, what medications are used in the treatment of pneumonia?

_____

_____

_____

II. Comprehension of the text

Directions: According to the following conversation and complete the sentences.

1. According to the article, the risk factor of pneumonia is _____.

　　A. drug addiction　　　　B. smoking　　　　C. ageing

笔记

2. People with pneumonia should not _____.

  A. eat too much fat and lard

  B. eat unhealthily

  C. drink boiled water

3. Which drug can be used to treat bronchitis?

  A. Erythromycin   B. Amoxicillin   C. Dolan tin

4. Which of the following drugs can not treat pneumonia?

  A. Streptomycin   B. Penicillin   C. Cimetidine

5. Which of the following is the symptom of patient with pneumonia？

  A. having a fever   B. flushing   C. breathing slowly

ER-4-13
扫一扫 答案
"晓"

Conversation 2

Treatment of Patients with Chronic Obstructive Pulmonary Disease

Two doctors talk about chronic obstructive pulmonary disease.

ER-4-14
扫一扫 听一
听

ER-4-15
扫一扫 知情
节

Doctor A: Today we are discussing the topic of chronic obstructive pulmonary disease.

Doctor B: Chronic obstructive pulmonary disease, or COPD, is a life-threatening condition commonly caused by years of smoking.

Doctor A: Yes. Over time, smoking interferes with the natural exchange of oxygen and carbon dioxide in the lungs.

Doctor B: And COPD is not curable.

Doctor A: But treatment can extend a patient's life. We often treat it with steroids. Now, a study shows that low doses of the medicine given by mouth are equal to, or better than, a heavy dose administered into the blood.

Doctor B: And the study found that those who received lower doses of steroids by mouth spent less time in the hospital.

Doctor A: Can you tell me what's the cause of the chronic obstructive pulmonary disease?

Doctor B: The most common cause is long-term smoking or years of breathing other people's smoke.

Doctor A: What are the symptoms of the patients with chronic obstructive pulmonary disease?

Doctor B: Chronic obstructive pulmonary disease includes emphysema and chronic bronchitis, as well as asthmatic bronchitis. One sign of it is a wheezing sound when the person breathes. Another symptom is a cough that produces yellow mucus and does not go away.

Doctor A: You are right. COPD blocks airflow in the lungs. And patients have to think about their breathing. They also have to exercise. And they have to learn to calm themselves, especially when they are short of breath.

Doctor B: First of all the patient should give up smoking, and have a healthy lifestyle, but also strengthen exercise. In addition, the patient needs to use the bronchial dilation.

(295 words)

笔 记

Words in Focus

curable /ˈkjʊrəbl/	*adj.*	可治愈的
steroid /ˈsterɔid/	*n.*	类固醇
emphysema /ˌemfiˈsiːmə/	*n.*	肺气肿
wheeze /wiːz/	*v.*	发出呼哧呼哧的喘息声
mucus /ˈmjuːkəs/	*n.*	黏液
airflow /ˈeəflou/	*n.*	空气的流动
dilation /daiˈleiʃn/	*n.*	膨胀，扩张，扩大

ER-4-16
扫一扫 读一读

Useful Expressions

chronic obstructive pulmonary disease	慢性阻塞性肺疾病
chronic bronchitis	慢性支气管炎
asthmatic bronchitis	喘息性支气管炎
go away	离开

ER-4-17
扫一扫 看一看

I. Free talk

Directions: Work in pairs and discuss the following questions after learning to the dialogue two.

1. According to the article, what is the most common cause of chronic obstructive pulmonary disease?

_____

_____

2. According to the article, what drugs are used in the treatment of chronic obstructive pulmonary disease?

_____

_____

II. Comprehension of the text

Directions: According to the conversation and complete the sentences

1. Which of the following is not a symptom of patients with chronic obstructive pulmonary disease?

   A. dyspnea

   B. anorexia

   C. sputum volume reduction

2. If a person has chronic obstructive pulmonary disease, can he be cured?

   A. yes　　　　　　　B. no　　　　　　　C. uncertain

3. Which one of the following options is something you can do when suffering from chronic obstructive pulmonary disease?

   A. smoking　　　　B. drinking alcohol　　　　C. doing more exercise

4. Which of the following can lead to chronic obstructive pulmonary disease?

   A. unreasonable way of life　　B. obesity　　　　C. smoking

5. People at which age are most likely to have chronic obstructive pulmonary disease?

   A. 20　　　　　　　B. 30　　　　　　　C. 50

ER-4-18
扫一扫 答案
"晓"

笔记

51

Part Ⅲ　Reading

Text A

ER-4-19
扫一扫 听一
听

ER-4-20
扫一扫 知情
节

> This article has introduced the death trend of lung cancer in recent years and the causes of lung cancer. It also briefly illustrates the formation of the disease and basic measures taken to deal with it.
>
> **Pre-reading**
> 1. What is the influence of lung cancer?
> 2. How to prevent the lung cancer?

Lung Cancer

The death rate due to cancer of the lungs has increased more than 800 percent in males and has more than doubled in females during the last 25 years. It is considerably higher in urban and industrial areas than in rural districts. There are many possible causes, but it is still controversial which are most blameworthy. Those factors which have been mentioned most frequently are the presence of foreign particles and other irritants in the air (smoke particles, smog, exhaust fumes), and the smoking of cigarettes and cigars.

Numerous studies have demonstrated a striking correlation between the death rate from lung cancer and smoking habits. Among heavy smokers 21 to 30 cigarettes per day —the mortality rate from lung cancer is nearly 17 times the rate from nonsmokers. It is expected the death rate among women will increase as the present high rate of smoking among women has its effect.

Sometimes cases of lung cancer are discovered at the time an x-ray is taken for the purpose of detecting tuberculosis. Too often, however, a current emphasis upon the danger of exposure to radiation from X-ray machines can frighten people away from routine chest X-rays and thus prevent an early diagnosis of lung cancer. Early detection is absolutely essential if any possibility of cure is to be maintained. People with skills operate modern X-ray machine. It takes small risk to the people who are over 40 years old. So the risk would be much more than offset by the advantages of discovering a tumor while it is small enough to be completely removed.

A common form of lung cancer is bronchogenic carcinoma, so-called because the malignancy originates in a bronchus. The tumor may grow until the bronchus is blocked, cutting off the supply of air to that lung. The lung then collapses, and the secretions trapped in the lung spaces become infected, with a resulting pneumonia or the formation of a lung abscess. Such a lung cancer can also spread to cause secondary growths in the lymph nodes of the chest and neck as well as in the brain and other parts of the body. The only treatment that offers a possibility of cure, before secondary growths have had time to form, is to remove the lung completely. This operation is called pneumonectomy.

Malignant tumors of the stomach, the breast, the prostate gland and other organs may spread

笔记

to the lungs, causing secondary growths.

(403 words)

Words in Focus

blameworthy /ˈbleɪmwɜːði/	*adj.*	应受谴责的；该受责备的
bronchus /ˈbrɑŋkəs/	*n.*	支气管
irritant /ˈɪrɪtənt/	*adj.*	刺激的；刺激性的
smog /smɑːg/	*n.*	烟雾
secretion /sɪˈkriʃən/	*n.*	分泌；分泌物
abscess /ˈæbˈsɛs/	*n.*	脓肿；脓疮
mortality /mɔˈtæliti/	*n.*	死亡率；必死性
pneumonectomy /ˌnjuməˈnɛktəmi/	*n.*	肺切除术
tuberculosis /tuˈbɜkjəˈlosis/	*n.*	肺结核
malignant /məˈlignənt/	*adj.*	恶性的；有害的
correlation /ˌkɔrəˈleiʃən/	*n.*	相关；关联

ER-4-21
扫一扫 读一读

ER-4-22
扫一扫 看一看

Useful Expressions

exposure to radiation	接触放射线
bronchogenic carcinoma	支气管癌
lymph node	淋巴结
prostate gland	前列腺

Post-reading

I. Comprehension of the text

Choose the best answer to complete each sentence with the information from the text.

1. Which is the most blameworthy cause of lung cancer?

    A. Smoking.

    B. Environmental pollution.

    C. It is still controversial.

2. What's the relationship between smoking and lung cancer mortality？

    A. Smoking can reduce the lung cancer mortality.

    B. The more one smokes, the bigger chances of getting lung cancer he will have.

    C. Lung cancer mortality is not related to smoking.

3. What hinders the early diagnosis of lung cancer？

    A. Medical technology is not developed.

    B. It is not necessary to pay attention to it.

    C. People think it's very dangerous to be exposed to X-ray.

4. In which situation, pneumonectomy can be carried out?

    A. The patient's cardiopulmonary compensatory ability is poor.

    B. After anti-tuberculosis treatment, the patient's condition still worsens.

    C. In other parts of the patient's lung appear new infiltrations STD focuses.

5. According to the passage, how a primary lung cancer patient may be cured?

    A. Use chemotherapy and radiotherapy or combination therapy.

    B. Give priority to chemotherapy, and then choose one among palliative radiation therapy,

笔记

immunotherapy, cortical steroids, analgesics and antibiotic treatment according to the condition.

C. Remove the lung completely before the cancer cells spread elsewhere.

II. Vocabulary activities

Find a word or phrase from the box below to complete each sentence. There are more words and phrases than you need to fill in all the sentences. Change word forms where necessary.

bronchogenic	correlation	emphasis	blameworthy	abscess
irritant	lymph	controversial	essential	industrial
malignancy	diagnosis	offset	collapse	

1. Tocqueville, seldom in good health, lived on his nerves, working in bursts followed by frequent _____.

2. In the 18th and 19th centuries, the _____ Revolution transformed the socioeconomic texture of Britain.

3. Loss of appetite or anorexia is often associated with cachexia, especially cachexia of _____.

4. The struggle to improve efficiency and cut costs is a constant _____ in labor-management relations.

5. Doctors not familiar with ciguatera sometimes mistakenly give a _____ of chronic fatigue syndrome.

6. In Ms. Price's case, the chairman said there was no evidence that she had done anything wrong in her role as head of PE and pastoral care, and the panel had found no kind of _____ conduct.

7. Raven was also first to find a strong _____ between insulin resistance and heart attacks.

8. And when breast cancers did occur they tended to be larger tumours spreading to _____ nodes.

9. The European Parliament has voted for sweeping reforms of the _____ EU Common Fisheries Policy.

10. Davis' five-under round came despite having overnight hospital treatment to remove a mouth _____.

III. Check your comprehension

Read the following statements and then decide whether each of them is true or false based on the information from the text. Write T for true and F for false in the space provided.

_____ 1. Lung cancer can cause problems in various parts of the body and it can be caused by other physical diseases.

_____ 2. The tumor is so big that it blocks up the bronchus. It will block the exchange of gases.

_____ 3. The pneumonectomy is the only treatment that can cure the patient.

_____ 4. Long-term smoking must cause lung cancer.

ER-4-23
扫一扫 答案
"晓"

ER-4-24
扫一扫 练一练

笔记

IV. Supplementary

Text B

This article introduces the history, the classification and prevention of silicosis. It especially focuses on its signs and symptoms. It also involves some disorders caused by silicosis.

Pre-reading

1. What is the connection between silicosis and environment?
2. People in which workplace have more possibility to get silicosis?

ER-4-25
扫一扫 听一听

ER-4-26
扫一扫 知情节

Silicosis

Silicosis (previously miner's phthisis, grinder's asthma, potter's rot and other occupation-related names) is a form of occupational lung disease caused by inhalation of crystalline silica dust, and is marked by inflammation and scarring in the form of nodular lesions in the upper lobes of the lungs. It is a type of pneumoconiosis.

Silicosis resulted in 46,000 deaths globally in 2013 down from 55,000 deaths in 1990. The name silicosis (from the Latin silex, or flint) was originally used in 1870 by Achille Visconti (1836-1911), prosector in the Ospedale Maggiore of Milan. The recognition of respiratory problems from breathing in dust dates to ancient Greeks and Romans. Agricola, in the mid-16th century, wrote about lung problems from dust inhalation in miners. In 1713, Bernardino Ramazzini noted asthmatic symptoms and sand-like substances in the lungs of stone cutters. With industrialization, as opposed to hand tools, came increased production of dust. The pneumatic hammer drill was introduced in 1897 and sandblasting was introduced in about 1904, both significantly contributing to the increased prevalence of silicosis.

Classification of silicosis is made according to the disease's severity (including radiographic pattern), onset, and rapidity of progression. These include chronic simple silicosis, accelerate silicosis, complicated silicosis and acute silicosis.

Because chronic silicosis is slow to develop, signs and symptoms may not appear until years after exposure. Signs and symptoms include:

- Dyspnea (shortness of breath) exacerbated by exertion
- Cough, often persistent and sometimes severe
- Fatigue
- Tachypnea (rapid breathing) which is often labored
- Loss of appetite and weight loss (Anorexia)
- Chest pain
- Fever
- Gradual dark shallow rifts in nails eventually leading to cracks as protein fibers within nail beds are destroyed.

In advanced cases, the following may also occur:

- Cyanosis (blue skin)
- Cor pulmonale (right ventricle heart disease)

笔记

● Respiratory insufficiency

Patients with silicosis are particularly susceptible to tuberculosis (TB) infection—known as silicotuberculosis. The reason for the increased risk—3 fold increased incidence—is not well understood. It is thought that silica damages pulmonary macrophages, inhibiting their ability to kill mycobacteria. Even workers with prolonged silica exposure, but without silicosis, are at a similarly increased risk for TB.

Pulmonary complications of silicosis also include Chronic Bronchitis and airflow limitation (indistinguishable from that caused by smoking), non-tuberculous Mycobacterium infection, fungal lung infection, compensatory emphysema, and pneumothorax. There are some data revealing an association between silicosis and certain autoimmune diseases, including nephritis, Scleroderma, and Systemic Lupus Erythematosus, especially in acute or accelerated silicosis.

The best way to prevent silicosis is to identify work-place activities that produce respirable crystalline silica dust and then to eliminate or control the dust. Water spray is often used where dust emanates. Dust can also be controlled through dry air filtering.

(444 words)

Words in Focus

pneumoconiosis /ˌnjuməˌkoniˈosɪs/	n.	尘肺病，肺尘埃沉着病
cyanosis /ˌsaiəˈnosis/	n.	苍白病，黄萎病
asthmatic /æsˈmætik/	adj.	气喘的，似患气喘的
prosector /prə(ʊ)ˈsektə/	n.	解剖员
accelerated /əkˈseləreitid/	v.	加速，促进
complicated /ˈkɑmplikeitid/	adj.	难懂的，复杂的
acute /əˈkjut/	adj.	急性的，敏锐的
dyspnea /dispˈniə/	n.	呼吸困难
fatigue /fəˈtig/	n.	疲乏，杂役
ventricle /ˈvɛntrikl/	n.	心室，脑室
macrophage /ˈmækrəˈfeidʒ/	n.	巨噬细胞，大噬细胞
carcinogenic /ˌkɑsinəˈdʒɛnik/	adj.	致癌的，致癌物的

Useful Expressions

shortness of breathe	气促，呼吸浅短
pulmonary edema	肺水肿
crystalline silica	结晶二氧化硅，石英
nodular lesion	结节性病灶

Post-reading

I. Comprehension of the text

I) Answer the following questions with the information from the text.

1. From this passage, people in which working condition have higher chance of having silicosis?

2. In paragraph 2, it introduces us the history about silicosis. What appears to increase the prevalence of silicosis?

3. What are the signs and symptoms when silicosis attacks?

4. In order to keep the workers healthy, can you give some advice to factory managers?

ER-4-27
扫一扫 读一读

ER-4-28
扫一扫 看一看

笔记

II) Read the following statements and then decide whether each of them is true or false based on the information from the text. Write T for true and F for false in the space provided.

_____1. People who inhales a lot of free silica dust in short term may get silicosis years after.

_____2. Pulmonary tuberculosis concurrent rate increases with the progress of the phase silicosis.

_____3. We can clearly understand the reason why the incidence and risk of silicosis are increasing.

_____4. People attached great importance to silicosis a long time ago.

II. Vocabulary activities

Find a word or phrase from the box below to complete each sentence. There are more words and phrases than you need to fill in all the sentences. Change word forms where necessary.

ingest	exposure to	clinically	acute	distinguishable
eliminate	asthmatic	alleviate	possible	prolong
scarring	pneumatic	lead to	unremarkable	

1. With the world economy wobbling, this _____ conflict is something Thailand could badly do without.

2. He said Ms. Bending, who was _____, may have suffered a severe asthma attack.

3. Some fertility experts fear the guidelines may not _____ changes because they are not binding.

4. Not surprisingly, businesses continue to grapple with how to _____, understand, and operationalize Big Data.

5. Like many of us, her main _____ that city's rich culture is through friends, food and music.

6. Seth Godin wrote in his book Purple Cow that remarkable things will succeed against _____ things.

7. Nurturing others — raising children, teaching, caring for animals — helps to _____ loneliness.

8. The men are all _____ depressed because their girlfriends' "favorite mascot" strategy works every year.

9. The wide-body, twin-engine jet relies on a complex network of electrical systems rather than traditional _____ systems.

10. Its cities are generally beautiful and preserved, because they avoided the _____ of World War II.

III. Supplementary

ER-4-29
扫一扫 答案
"晓"

ER-4-30
扫一扫 练一
练

Part Ⅳ   Writing

Writing a Discharge Record

Instructions:

Hospital discharge record is a summary of hospitalized patients with diagnosis and treatment for the convenience of future reference.

笔记

In order to prove that one's discharge record is authentic, the following should be done and taken into consideration:

1. Name of hospital, patient's name, division, surgery, admission number of patient, etc.
2. Date of admission, date of discharge and length of hospitalization.
3. Admission condition, diagnosis and treatment after hospitalization, change of condition.
4. When discharged from hospital, degree of recovery, signs and symptoms of sequela etc.
5. Discharge diagnosis.
6. Doctor's advice: including considerations and suggestions, name and number of the drug as well as the dosage and usage.
7. Discharge record completed within 24 hours after patient's discharge from hospital. Be concise, to the point, and covers all the main information, such as hospital, CT, MRI, X-ray, etc.

Examples:

出院记录

昌邑市宋庄卫生院

科别：呼吸科   门诊号：*636   住院号：45

姓名：董明东   性别：男   年龄：24 岁

入院日期：2011 年 6 月 14 日   出院日期：2011 年 7 月 18 日

住院天数：35 天

入院情况：因间断咳嗽咳痰 3 个月余，加重 3 天入院。全身皮肤黏膜无黄染及出血点，浅表淋巴结未触及肿大。耳鼻无异常分泌物。血常规检查正常。

入院诊断：Ⅲ型肺结核

诊疗经过：入院后完善相关辅助检查进一步明确诊断，胸片右上中肺野示斑片状密度不均匀，查痰及培养显示阳性。治疗效果明显，继以抗炎、抗痨等治疗，好转出院。

出院诊断：Ⅲ型肺结核

出院医嘱：1. 注意休息，避免受凉，控制饮食。

     2. 继续服药。

     3. 不适随诊。

上级医师 / 住院医师签名：＿＿＿＿＿＿

Examples:

The discharge record

Song zhuang Health Center of Chang yi City

Division: Pneumology Department Patient No:*636 AD: 45

Name: Dong Mingdong   Sex: Male Age: 24

Date of Admission: June 14, 2011 Date of Discharge: July 18, 2011

Length of stay: 35 days

Admission condition: cough and expectorate discontinuously for 3 months, aggravate 3 days ago; There was no jaundice, no purpura on the skin and membtane, and the lymphnodes were not palpable; no abnormal discharge from ear and nose; blood routine examination normal.

Diagnosis after hospitalization: III tuberculosis

Treatment procedure: diagnosis clarified after related auxiliary examination, chest radiograph shows spots in the upper right lung are in inhomogeneous density. Phlegm and sputum culture are positive.

Treatment effect is obvious after anti-inflammatory treatment and antituberculosis treatment.

Discharge Diagnosis: Ⅲ tuberculosis

Doctor's advice:

1. Have a good rest; avoid catching cold and control the diet.

2. Continue to take medicine.

3. See the doctor when feeling sick.

Signature: _____

Practice :

出院记录

科别：呼吸　　　　病人姓名：胡志远

性别：男　　　　年龄：72　　　　　　职业：离休干部

入院日期：2011 年 10 月 10 日　　　　出院日期：2011 年 12 月 15 日

入院情况（包括检验异常结果等）：因慢性咳嗽、咳痰 16 年，发作性胸骨后闷痛 1 年余，加重伴发热 2 天。血常规检查异常。X 线胸透：两肺透亮度增加，肺纹理增粗、紊乱，呈索条状。心电图：窦性心动过速，电轴左偏，TI、aVL、V5、V6 低平。

诊疗经过：入院后给予药物治疗，2 周后感染控制，咳嗽、咳痰减轻，体温恢复正常，并给予控制饮食和其他药物治疗，患者一般活动无胸痛及气促。

出院情况（包括主要化验结果）：咳嗽、咳痰减轻，无胸痛，病情稳定。心电图基本正常。

入院诊断：

（1）慢性支气管炎急性发作期，阻塞性肺气肿

（2）冠心病，劳累性心绞痛，稳定型

（3）高脂血症

（4）非胰岛素依赖型糖尿病

（5）前列腺良性增生

（6）全口义齿

出院诊断：

（1）慢性支气管炎急性发作期，阻塞性肺气肿

（2）冠心病，劳累性心绞痛，稳定型

（3）高脂血症

（4）非胰岛素依赖型糖尿病

（5）前列腺良性增生

（6）全口义齿

出院医嘱：

1．坚持饮食疗法，适当活动，防止感冒

2．按时吃药

3．2 周后门诊随访

（复诊时携带出院记录）

医师签字：_____

ER-4-31
扫一扫 答案
"晓"

笔记

Part Ⅴ　Enriching your word power

1. bronch(o)- 支气管
   bronchodilator /ˌbrɒŋkəʊdaiˈleitə/ 支气管扩张药
   bronchopneumonia /ˌbrɒŋkə(ʊ)njuːˈməuniə/ 支气管肺炎
2. capn(o)-; carb(o)- 二氧化碳，碳
   capnometer /ˈkæpnəumitə/ 二氧化碳测定器
   carbohemia /kɑːbəˈhiːmiə/ 碳酸血症，二氧化碳血症
3. laryng(o)- 喉
   laryngitis /ˌlærinˈdʒaitis/ 喉炎
   laryngostenosis /ləˈriŋəʊstiˈnəusis/ 喉狭窄
4. nas(o)-; rhin(o)- 鼻
   nasogastric /neizəʊˈgæstrik/ 鼻饲的
   rhinolaryngology /rainəʊlærinˈgɒlədʒi/ 鼻喉科学
5. pharyng(o)- 咽
   pharyngodynia /fæˈriŋɔdiniə/ 咽痛；咽部疼痛
   pharyngotonsillitis /færiŋəʊtɒnsiˈlaitis/ 咽扁桃体炎
6. pneum(o)-; pneumon(o)- 气，肺
   pneumonectasis /njuːməˈnektəsis/ 肺气肿
   pneumohemothorax /njuːməuhiːməˈθɔːræks/ 血气胸
7. trache(o)- 气管
   tracheobronchitis /treikiəubrɒŋˈkaitis/ 气管支气管炎
   tracheotomy /ˌtrækiˈɒtəmi/ 气管切开术
8. pnea- 呼吸
   dyspnea /disˈpniːə/ 呼吸困难
   bradypnea /bˈrædipniə/ 呼吸迟缓
9. pleur(o)- 胸膜
   pleura /ˈpluərə/ 肋膜；胸膜
   pleurocentesis /pluərəsenˈtiːsis/ 胸腔穿刺术
10. pulmon(o)- 肺
    pulmonology /pʌlˈmənɒlədʒi/ 肺脏学
    pulmonohepatic /pʌlmənəuhˈpætik/ 肺肝的
11. sinus(o)- 窦
    sinusotomy /ˈsainəsətəmi/ 窦切开术
    sinusitis /ˌsainəˈsaitis/ 窦炎
12. thorac(o)-; pector(o)-; steth(o)- 胸
    thoracocentesis /θɔːrəkəˈsəntizis/ 同 thoracentesis 胸腔穿刺术
    pectoralgia /pektəˈrældʒə/ 胸痛
    stethomyositis /sˈtetəmaiəsaitis/ 胸肌炎

笔记

Part Ⅵ Exercise

Directions: *In this section, only one of the following options is correct, please choose.*

（王利亚　吕小君）

ER-4-32
扫一扫 看一
看

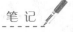

笔记

Unit 5
Digestive Department

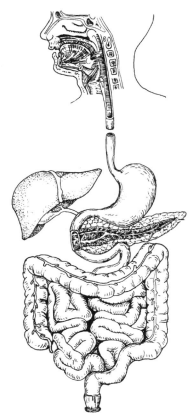

Fig. 5-1   digestive department

Eat breakfast like a king, lunch like a prince and dinner like a pauper.

早餐吃得像国王，午餐像王子，晚餐像乞丐。

——Adelle Davis（阿戴尔·戴维斯）

Learning Objectives

Skill focus

1. *Get basic ideas of hepatitis and pancreatitis.*

2. *Understand conversations between nurse and patient during the gastroscopy procedure.*

3. *Learn the basic nursing interventions related to peptic ulcer.*

Language focus

1. *Be familiar with the words, phrases related to the disease of digestive tract.*

2. *Be able to write a referral.*

笔记

Part Ⅰ　Listening

This section is designed to test your ability to understand spoken English in nursing or medical contexts. You will hear a selection of recorded materials and you must answer the questions that accompany them. There are TWO parts in this section, Part A and Part B.

Part A

Words in Focus

gastroscopy /gæs'trɒskəpi/	*n.*	胃镜检查法
endoscope /'endəskoup/	*n.*	内窥镜
flexible /'flɛksibəl/	*adj.*	灵活的；柔韧的
swallow /'swɑ:lou/	*vt.& vi.*	吞，咽；忍耐，忍受
sedative /'sɛdətiv/	*n.*	镇静剂，止痛药
injection /in'dʒɛkʃən/	*n.*	注射；注射剂
drowsy /'drauzi/	*adj.*	昏昏欲睡的；沉寂的
anesthetic /,ænis'θɛtik/	*n.*	麻醉剂，麻醉药
biopsy /'baiɑ:psi/	*n.*	活组织检查，活体检视
pathology /pə'θɑ:lədʒi/	*n.*	病理（学）

ER-5-1
扫一扫 读一读

ER-5-2
扫一扫 看一看

Useful Expressions

as...as	与……一样；相似的
make an appointment	预约
biopsy sample	活检组织，活检样本

Text

Directions: *You're going to hear one conversation at the end of the passage, one or more questions will be asked about what was said, decide which the best answer is.*

Background:

　　Mr. Yang is going to have a check at the Department of Gastroenterology, the nurse will give him some instructions about gastroscopy preparation.

ER-5-3
扫一扫 听一听

Comprehension of the text

1. What does an endoscope look like? _____

　　A. thin and flexible　　　　B. as long as a finger　　　C. a long pipe

2. What should Mr. Yang do before having the gastroscopy? _____

　　A. Drink a lot of water.

　　B. Smoke as much as possible.

　　C. Empty the stomach.

3. Will Mr. Yang feel hurt during the test? _____

　　A. Yes, intense pain.

　　B. No, just a little uncomfortable.

　　C. No, a little pain.

ER-5-4
扫一扫 知情节

笔记

4. When is Mr. Yang supposed to come tomorrow? _____

    A. 7 a.m.   B. 8 a.m.   C. 8:30 a.m.

5. What will be sent to the pathology laboratory? _____

    A. blood sample   B. biopsy sample   C. tissue sample

Part B

Words in Focus

endoscopy /en'dɑːskəpi/	*n.*	内窥镜检查术
instrument /'ɪnstrəmənt/	*n.*	仪器
interior /ɪn'tɪriə(r)/	*n.*	内部；内心
surgery /'sɜːdʒəri/	*n.*	外科手术
anesthetize /'ənɛsθə,taɪz/	*v.*	使麻醉；使麻木
gastrointestinal /ˌɡæstroʊin'testinl/	*adj.*	胃与肠的
bladder /'blædə(r)/	*n.*	膀胱

Useful Expressions

depend on   随……而定；依赖

Text

Directions: *In this section you will hear a short passage, before listening you will have 5 seconds to read each of the questions which accompany it. While listening, answer each question by choosing A, B, or C. After listening, you will have 5 seconds to check your answer to each question.*

Background:

    This is an instruction of endoscope.

1. Endoscopy is a _____ procedure done with an instrument called an endoscope.

    A. medical   B. clinical   C. inflammatory

2. Looking with an endoscope is different from using _____, like x-rays and CT scans.

    A. blood tests   B. other tests   C. imaging tests

3. There are many different types of endoscope, and depending on _____ and the type of procedure.

    A. the symptoms   B. the site in the body   C. the pain

4. Most of endoscopes are like _____, hollow tubes.

    A. thin   B. thick   C. short

5. Endoscopes are different lengths and shapes. Some are stiff, while others are _____.

    A. flexible   B. soft   C. nimble

Part II Speaking

    This section is designed to test your speaking ability. After learning the following conversation A and B you will have the ability of speaking skill in medical and nursing working and try to do the following speaking tasks.

ER-5-5
扫一扫 读一读

ER-5-6
扫一扫 看一看

ER-5-7
扫一扫 听一听

ER-5-8
扫一扫 知情节

笔记

Conversation 1

Peptic Ulcer

The patient Mr. Li went to the hospital because of the stomach pain. The nurse Mrs. Gao asked him about his symptoms. The patient told the nurse that he had too much at supper yesterday evening and caused a pain in the abdomen at night.

Nurse:　Good afternoon. What seems to be your trouble?

Patient:　It's my stomach. I think probably I had too much at supper yesterday evening.

Nurse:　Can you tell me what you had for supper yesterday evening?

Patient:　Seafood, roast duck. Oh, a great variety of things, I can't remember them exactly.

Nurse:　Have you vomited?

Patient:　Yes, I have vomited three times and made several trips to the bathroom last night.

Nurse:　Have you got any pain?

Patient:　Yes, it is in the upper side of my abdomen.

Nurse:　What kind of pain is it?

Patient:　It's sort of burning pain.

Nurse:　How long have you had this pain?

Patient　I've had it for two years, but it's never been this bad before.

Nurse:　When do you feel the worst pain?

Patient　In the middle of the night.

Nurse:　Did the doctor give you a test sheet just now? You have to get your stools tested and take it to the laboratory. Wait for a while and pick up the report, and then bring it back to me.

Patient:　All right, nurse. I'll see you later.

Nurse:　See you later.

Patient:　Here' s my report, nurse.

Nurse:　Take the seat, please, don't worry, and let me have a look. According to your symptoms and result, it looks like you have peptic ulcer.

Patient:　Is it serious?

Nurse:　We shall have to take an x-ray picture of your stomach and intestines. You must notice diet.

Patient:　All right.

Nurse:　It will be worse after you eat spicy food or onions.

Patient:　OK, I will avoid them recently.

Nurse:　I do advise you to avoid oily food for the next few days.

Patient:　I will follow your advice. Thanks a lot.

Nurse:　You are welcome.

(365 words)

Words in Focus

seafood /'si,fud/	*n.*	海鲜
bathroom /'bæθru:m/	*n.*	厕所；卫生间
abdomen /'æbdəmən/	*n.*	腹部；腹腔

burning /ˈbɜːnɪŋ/	adj.	燃烧的
laboratory /ˈlæbrətɔːri/	n.	实验室
intestines /inˈtestinz/	n.	肠
spicy /ˈspaisi/	adj.	辛辣的；有刺激性的

Useful Expressions

roast duck	烤鸭
test sheet	化验单
stools test	粪便检验
peptic ulcer	消化性溃疡

I. Free talk

Directions: *Work in pairs and discuss the following questions after learning to the recording of Dialogue One.*

1. Discuss with your partner: what are the symptoms of this patient?

_____

_____

2. What is the matter with this patient according to the result?

_____

_____

II. Comprehension of the text

Directions: *According to the conversation and complete the sentences.*

1. Peptic ulcer will cause _____.

   A. abdomen pain   B. headache   C. toothache

2. _____ can help to identify peptic ulcers.

   A. Blood test   B. X-ray picture   C. Ultrasound

3. _____ is necessary for the patient according to the passage.

   A. Stools test   B. Urine test   C. Blood test

4. The symptoms of peptic ulcer will be worse after you eat _____ or onions.

   A. sweet food   B. salty food   C. spicy food

5. The patient of peptic ulcer have to avoid _____ diet.

   A. delicate   B. oily   C. insipid

Conversation 2

Health Education for Patients with Liver Cirrhosis

A primary nurse is going to give Mr. Wu, the patient with liver cirrhosis and abdominal dropsy a health education. What should the nurse do to help the patient?

Nurse:　Good morning, Mr. Wu. I'm your primary nurse. I'll give you a healthy education. Do you have any question?

Patient:　Oh! I still feel weak these days.

Nurse:　Don't worry, Mr. Wu. You should strengthen nutrition diet, as well as proper protein such as soy food supplement.

Patient:　Then I can rest assured. I've been feeling my appetite has been enhanced.

Nurse:　I'm glad to hear that. Are you still sick and vomit?

Patient: It's better than the other day.

Nurse: You don't have to worry, as long as you actively cooperate with our treatment and pay attention to the diet, it will certainly be improved.

Patient: I must cooperate. How about my skin and complexion?

Nurse: You look better today. I'll look for you on palpation.

Patient: OK.

Nurse: I press your abdomen, if you get a pain, tell me.

Patient: Oh, a bit of pain.

Nurse: You still have a little abdominal dropsy due to your liver disease.

Patient: So what should I do?

Nurse: You should pay attention to have a rest, to maintain the law of life, must not stay up late and strenuous exercise.

Patient: All right. What do I need to pay attention to in the diet?

Nurse: Eating high calorie, high protein, high vitamin, digestible food. You need low salt diet, avoid eating rough, hard, chewy foods, such as fried pasta, hard fruit.

Patient: OK, I'll remember these.

Nurse: Avoid spicy condiment, drinking or irritating food. A balanced diet with both drug and rest will help you recover as soon as possible.

Patient: Nice talking to you, I'll follow you.

(337 words)

ER-5-14
扫一扫 听一听

ER-5-15
扫一扫 知情节

ER-5-16
扫一扫 读一读

Words in Focus

primary /ˈpraɪməri/	adj.	首要的；主要的
strengthen /ˈstrɛŋkθən,ˈstrɛŋ-,ˈstrɛn-/	vt.	加强，巩固；勉励
appetite /ˈæpɪˌtaɪt/	n.	食欲，胃口
complexion /kəmˈplɛkʃən/	n.	肤色，面色，气色
strenuous /ˈstrɛnjuəs/	adj.	紧张的；费力的；热烈的
digestible /daɪˈdʒɛstəbəl, di-/	adj.	易消化的
irritating /ˈiriteitiŋ/	adj.	刺激性的
condiment /ˈkɑːndimənt/	n.	调味品；佐料

ER-5-17
扫一扫 看一看

Useful Expressions

primary nurse	责任护士
cooperate with	与……配合
abdominal dropsy	腹水

I. Free talk

Directions: Work in pairs and discuss the following questions after learning to the Dialogue Two.

1. Why does Mr. Wu have abdominal dropsy?

_____

_____

2. What does Mr. Wu need to pay attention to in the diet?

_____

_____

ER-5-18
扫一扫 答案
"晓"

笔记

II. Work in pairs.

Directions: *If you are a nurse to give a health education to a patient of liver cirrhosis, What would you say?*

Part III   Reading

Text A

ER-5-19
扫一扫 听一
听

ER-5-20
扫一扫 知情
节

> Hepatitis simply means an inflammation of the liver without pinpointing a specific cause. Hepatitis is most commonly caused by one type of virus. In its early stages, hepatitis may cause flu-like symptoms.
>
> **Pre-reading**
> 1. What is hepatitis?
> 2. What are the symptoms of acute and chronic hepatitis?

Hepatitis

Hepatitis is an inflammation of the liver, most commonly caused by a viral infection. Hepatitis may occur with limited or no symptoms, but often leads to jaundice (a yellow discoloration of the skin, mucous membrane, and conjunctiva), poor appetite, and malaise. Hepatitis is acute when it lasts less than six months and chronic when it persists longer.

Acute hepatitis can be self-limiting (healing on its own), can progress to chronic hepatitis, or, rarely, can cause acute liver failure. Chronic hepatitis may have no symptoms, or may progress over time to fibrosis (scarring of the liver) and cirrhosis (chronic liver failure).

Initial symptoms of acute hepatitis are non-specific and flu-like, may include malaise, muscle and joint aches, fever, nausea or vomiting, diarrhea, and headache. More specific symptoms are loss of appetite, aversion to smoking among smokers, dark urine, jaundice, and abdominal discomfort. Acute viral hepatitis is more likely to be asymptomatic in children. General symptoms may last for 1～2 weeks before jaundice develops, with the total illness lasting weeks.

Chronic hepatitis may cause nonspecific symptoms such as malaise, tiredness, and weakness, and often leads to no symptoms at all. It is commonly identified on blood tests performed either for screening or to evaluate nonspecific symptoms. The presence of jaundice indicates advanced liver damage. On physical examination there may be enlargement of the liver. Extensive damage to and scarring of liver leads to weight loss, easy bruising and bleeding, and accumulation of ascites (fluid in the abdomen).

Worldwide, viral hepatitis is the most common cause of liver inflammation. There are five main hepatitis viruses, referred to as types A, B, C, D and E. Hepatitis A and E are typically caused by ingestion of contaminated food or water. Hepatitis B, C and D usually occur as a result of parenteral contact with infected body fluids. Common modes of transmission for these viruses

笔记

include receipt of contaminated blood or blood products, invasive medical procedures using contaminated equipment and for hepatitis B transmission from mother to baby at birth, from family member to child, and also by sexual contact.

Hospitalization might be necessary when symptoms are severe or lab tests show liver damage. No medications are used to treat hepatitis A because it's a short-term infection that goes away on its own. Chronic hepatitis B can sometimes be treated using medications. The treatment of chronic hepatitis C has improved significantly with the use of two medications, interferon and ribavirin, often used in combination.

Patients with mild hepatitis may be treated at home. They should rest in bed until the fever and jaundice are gone and their appetite is normal. Kids with a lack of appetite should try smaller, more frequent meals and fluids that are high in calories. They should also eat healthy foods rich in protein and carbohydrates and drink plenty of water.

(482 words)

Words in Focus

hepatitis /ˌhɛpəˈtaitis/	*n.*	肝炎
inflammation /ˌinfləˈmeiʃən/	*n.*	炎症；燃烧
jaundice /ˈdʒɔndis, ˈdʒɑn-/	*n.*	黄疸病
mucous /ˈmjukəs/	*adj.*	黏液的，黏液覆盖的
membrane /ˈmɛmˌbrein/	*n.*	隔膜；(动、植物体内的)薄膜
conjunctiva /ˌkɒndʒʌŋkˈtaivə/	*n.*	(眼球)结膜
malaise /mæˈleiz, -ˈlɛz/	*n.*	萎靡不振；不适，不舒服
fibrosis /faiˈbrousis/	*n.*	纤维化，纤维症
cirrhosis /səˈrousis/	*n.*	肝硬化；硬变
solvents /ˈsɒlvənts/	*n.*	溶剂
asymptomatic /ˌesimptəˈmætik/	*adj.*	无临床症状的
scarring /ˈskɑriŋ/	*n.*	伤疤；瘢痕形成
bruising /ˈbruːziŋ/	*n.*	擦伤，挫伤
ascites /æˈsaitiːs/	*n.*	腹水

ER-5-21
扫一扫 读一读

ER-5-22
扫一扫 看一看

Useful Expressions

characterized by	以······为特征
poor appetite	食欲不振
toxic substances	有毒物质
dark urine	溺赤；小便黄赤

Post-reading

I. Comprehension of the text

Choose the best answer to complete each sentence with the information from the text.

1. Hepatitis is acute when it lasts less than _____ and chronic when it persists longer.

    A. one month   B. three months   C. six months

2. Acute hepatitis can be self-limiting (healing on its own), can progress to _____, or, rarely, can cause acute liver failure.

    A. hepatitis virus   B. chronic hepatitis   C. jaundice

笔记

3. Hepatitis B, C and D usually occur as a result of parenteral contact with _____ body fluids.

    A. infectant   B. infected   C. infections

4. Hospitalization might be necessary when symptoms are severe or lab tests show liver damage.

    _____

    A. Yes   B. No   C. Not mentioned

5. Chronic hepatitis may cause nonspecific symptoms such as malaise, _____, and weakness, and often leads to no symptoms at all.

    A. tiredness   B. vomiting   C. headache

II. Check your vocabulary

Find a word or phrase from the box below to complete each sentence. Change word forms where necessary.

persist	enlargement	define	harmful	cause
evaluate	identify	extensive	specific	advance

1. Hepatitis is a medical condition _____ by the inflammation of the liver.
2. Hepatitis is acute when it lasts less than six months and chronic when it _____ longer.
3. _____ symptoms of this baby included: fever, lung infection and anemia.
4. According to the National Cancer Institute(NCI), common symptoms of HL include the _____ of lymph nodes, spleen, fever, weight loss.
5. It is _____ to the liver to have quantities of alcohol frequently.
6. Heavy drinking will _____ high blood pressure.
7. Scientists claim to have _____ chemicals produced by certain plants which have powerful cancer-fighting function.
8. The patients were followed-up every 3 months for 1 year to _____ the clinical symptoms.
9. Most had _____ damage in eyes, and some had such limited vision.
10. The presence of jaundice indicates _____ liver damage.

III. Supplementary

Text B

ER-5-23
扫一扫 答案
"晓"

ER-5-24
扫一扫 练一
练

ER-5-25
扫一扫 听一
听

> Pancreatitis is an inflammatory process in which pancreatic enzymes auto digest the gland. Pancreatitis can be acute or chronic. Either form is serious and can lead to complications. In severe cases, bleeding, infection, and permanent tissue damage may occur.
>
> **Pre-reading**
> 1. What is pancreatitis?
> 2. What are the symptoms of acute pancreatitis?

ER-5-26
扫一扫 知情
节

笔记

Pancreatitis

Pancreatitis is a condition characterized by inflammation of the pancreas. It is a condition that may be mild and self-limiting, though it can also lead to severe complications that can be life-threatening. It can be an acute (short-term) or chronic (long-term) condition.

The causes of pancreatitis include: alcohol consumption, gallstones, high triglyceride levels, abdominal injury or surgery, certain medications, exposure to certain chemicals, smoking, family history of pancreatitis, cystic fibrosis and pancreatic cancer.

Acute pancreatitis generally develops suddenly, and it is usually a short-term (a few days to weeks) illness that typically resolves with appropriate medical management. The acute form of pancreatitis, in its most severe form, can have deleterious effects on many other body organs, including the lungs and kidneys.

Chronic pancreatitis, which typically develops after multiple episodes of acute pancreatitis, is a long-term condition that can last for months or even several years.

Pancreatitis causes upper abdominal pain which can range from mild to severe. The pain may come on suddenly or it may develop gradually. Often, the pain will start or worsen after eating, which can also occur with gallbladder or ulcer pain. Abdominal pain tends to be the hallmark of acute pancreatitis. People with acute pancreatitis usually feel very ill. In chronic pancreatitis, abdominal pain also can be present, but it is often not as severe, and some people may not have any pain at all.

There are a number of tests that alone, or in combination, will help establish the diagnosis of pancreatitis. Blood tests, such as liver and kidney function tests, tests for infection, or tests for anemia. Imaging studies. A CT (computed tomography) scan of the abdomen may be ordered to visualize the pancreas and to evaluate the extent of inflammation. Ultrasound imaging can be used to look for gallstones and abnormalities of the biliary system. Because ultrasound imaging does not emit radiation, this modality is frequently the initial imaging test obtained in cases of pancreatitis.

The following are some necessary nursing interventions for pancreatitis. Investigate verbal reports of pain, noting specific location and intensity (0～10 scale). Note factors that aggravate and relieve pain. Maintain bed-rest. Provide quiet, restful environment. Promote position of comfort on one side with knees flexed, sitting up and leaning forward. Reduces abdominal pressure and tension, providing some measure of comfort and pain relief, such as back rub, encourage relaxation techniques(guided imagery). Administer analgesics in timely manner(smaller, more frequent doses). Monitor serum glucose. Resume oral intake with clear liquids and advance diet slowly to provide high-protein, high-carbohydrate diet, when indicated. Advising the patient to avoid high fat diet and overeating, alternate work with rest, stop smoking and refrain from drinking.

(445 words)

Words in Focus

pancreatitis /ˌpænkriə'taitis/	*n.*	胰腺炎
characterized /'kærəktə,raizd/	*adj.*	具有特征的
pancreas /'pæŋkriəs, 'pæn-/	*n.*	胰，胰腺
abdominal /æb'dɑːminl/	*adj.*	腹部的
hormones /'hɔːmoun/	*n.*	荷尔蒙，激素

笔记

ER-5-27
扫一扫 读一读

ER-5-28
扫一扫 看一看

enzymes /ˈenzaimz/	n.	酶
metabolism /miˈtæbəˌlizəm/	n.	新陈代谢；代谢作用
deleterious /ˌdeləˈtiəriəs/	adj.	有害的；有毒的
episodes /ˈepisoudz/	n.	插曲，片断
gallstones /ˈgɔːlstounz/	n.	胆（结）石
triglyceride /traiˈglisəˌraid/	n.	甘油三酸酯
gallbladder /ˈgɔːlˌblædə/	n.	胆囊
visualize /ˈviʒuəˌlaiz/	vt.	使可见
modality /mouˈdæliti/	n.	方式，形式，模式

Useful Expressions

have ... effect on	对……有影响
multiple episodes	多个事件
break down	分解

Post-reading

I. Comprehension of the text

Ⅰ) Answer the following questions with the information from the text.

1. What is pancreatitis?

2. What are acute pancreatitis and chronic pancreatitis?

3. What are the causes of pancreatitis?

4. What are the signs and symptoms of pancreatitis?

5. How is pancreatitis diagnosed?

Ⅱ) Read the following statements and then decide whether each of them is true or false based on the information from the text. Write T for true and F for false in the space provided.

_____ 1. Pancreatitis can be an acute (short-term) or chronic (long-term) condition.

_____ 2. Chronic pancreatitis can have deleterious effects on many other body organs, including the lungs and kidneys.

_____ 3. The pain of pancreatitis always come on suddenly.

_____ 4. Ultrasound imaging does emit radiation.

II. Check your vocabulary

Find a word or phrase from the box below to complete each sentence. Change word forms where necessary.

| release | exposure | establish | situate | multiple |
| regulate | typical | severe | range from | in combination with |

1. Most villages are _____ in the lower valleys, where the climate is milder.

2. Experts found it helps _____ blood circulation in humans.

3. The disease _____ manifested itself in a high fever and chest pains.

4. We have _____ solutions of this problem.

5. She has contracted a _____ fever.

6. A bottle of sleeping tablets will _____ you from your sufferings forever.

7. _____ to lead is known to damage the brains of young children.

笔记

8. Without it, symptoms can _____ digestive disorders to very serious illnesses including bowel cancer.

9. Artemisinin（青蒿素）, given _____ other drugs, is the most effective malaria treatment today.

10. Medical tests _____ that she was not their own child.

III. Supplementary

ER-5-29
扫一扫 答案
"晓

ER-5-30
扫一扫 练一
练

Part Ⅳ   Writing

Writing a Medical Referral Letter

Instructions:

A medical referral letter is sent from one physician to another when referring a patient for care. Most often the letter is sent from the patient's general practitioner or primary care physician to a specialist with a request for diagnosis or treatment of a patient. Writing a medical referral letter is up to each individual doctor, although some medical groups have templates to be followed.

How to Write Medical Referral Letters? You should take these in consideration.

Check to see if your hospital or medical group has a template or prompt sheet for medical referral letters. If so, fill in the template with the applicable patient information and medical history.

Open a text document to begin your letter. Format the letter using a standard business letter template in your word processing program. If you don't have a template simply format it as a business letter. Include the date, your address, the address of the doctor you're sending it to, then the body of the letter and your signature.

Include the patient's personal information and the referring doctor's contact information in the letter. Also include the reason for the referral. Specialists prefer referral letters to include a patient's medical history, any clinical findings, prior test results and any previous treatments.

Sentence Patterns:

A medical referral letter usually consists of the following parts:

1. **the heading** (medical referral letter)
2. **the body** (the main content of the referral)
3. **the signature** (handwritten or typed)

Sample:

转诊信

河北省肿瘤医院（机构名称）

　　现有病人 张雪 性别 _女_ 年龄 _40_ ，因病情需要，需转入贵单位，请予以接诊。

　　转诊原因：乳腺癌

转诊医生（签字）：王欣

河北承德乡镇医院（机构名称）

2015 年 5 月 1 日

笔记

Medical Referral Letter

Date: <u>May 1, 2015</u>

To: <u>Hebei Provincial Tumour Hospital</u> (transferred to the department)

Dear Dr,

This is refer that the patient (name) <u>Zhang Xue</u>, (gender)<u>female</u>, aged <u>40</u>, who needs to <u>be transferred to your hospital for further treatment.</u>

Provisional diagnosis: <u>mammary cancer.</u>

Your expert management would be highly appreciated.

Signature: <u>Wang Xin</u>

(Turn out department): <u>Chengde Country Hospital, Hebei</u>

Practice:

请以护士张艺为名，拟写一封转诊信，病人蔡伟，男，45 岁，因肾结石复发需转诊到肾病科就诊，联系人胡医生。

_____

_____

_____

_____

_____

_____

_____

_____

_____

_____

ER-5-31
扫一扫 答案
"晓"

Part Ⅴ   Enriching your word power

1.　esophag(o)　食管
　　esophagocele /iˈsɒfəgəusiːl/　食管突出；食管疝
　　esophagostenosis /iːsɒfeigəstiˈnəusis/　食管狭窄

2.　gastr(o)　胃
　　gastrocolitis /ˈgæstrəukəlaitiz/　胃结肠炎
　　gastroscope /ˈgæstrəskəup/　胃窥镜

3.　duoden(o)　十二指肠
　　duodenoscopy /djuədiˈnəskəpi/　十二指肠镜检查
　　duodenoenterostomy /djuːədinəuntəˈrɒstəmi/　十二指肠小肠造口术

4.　enter(o)　肠，小肠
　　gastroenteritis /ˌgæstrəuˌentəˈraitis/　肠杆菌属
　　enterokinesia /entərəukaiˈniːsiə/　肠动，肠蠕动

5.　col(o); colon(o)　结肠
　　colocecostomy /kəuləuseˈkɒstəmi/ 同 cecocolostomy　结肠盲肠吻合术
　　colonitis /kɒləˈnaitis/　结肠炎

笔记

6.　rect(o); proct(o)　　　　　　　　　　　　　　　直肠
　　rectoclysis /'rektəukləsis/ 同 proctoclysis　　直肠滴注法
　　rectocele /'rektəsi:l/　　　　　　　　　　　脱肛（直肠向阴道突出）
　　proctitis /prɒk'taitis/　　　　　　　　　　直肠炎
7.　splen(o)　　　　　　　　　　　　　　　　脾
　　splenomegaly /,spli:nəu'megəli/ 同 splenomegalia　脾（肿）大
　　splenorrhagia /sple'nɔ:rædʒə/　　　　　　脾出血
8.　hepat(o)　　　　　　　　　　　　　　　肝
　　hepatomegaly /hepətəu'megəli/　　　　　肝肿大
　　hepatitis /,hepə'taitis/　　　　　　　　　肝炎
9.　bil(i); chol(e)　　　　　　　　　　　　　胆汁
　　bilirubin /,bili'ru:bɪn/　　　　　　　　　胆红素
　　cholecystectomy /,kɒlisis'tektəmi/　　　　胆囊切除术
　　cholelithiasis /kɒlili'θaiəsis/　　　　　　胆石症
10.　pancreat(o)　　　　　　　　　　　　　胰（腺）
　　pancreatolith /pæŋkri'ætəliθ/　　　　　　胰石
　　pancreatolysis /pæŋkriə'tɒləsis/ 同 pancreolysis　胰组织破坏
11.　abdomin(o);lapar(o); celi(o)　　　　　　腹
　　abdominocentesis /æb,dɒminəsen'ti:sis/　　腹腔穿刺术
　　laparoscopy /,læpə'rɒskəpi/　　　　　　腹腔镜检查
12.　peritone(o)　　　　　　　　　　　　　腹膜，腹腔
　　peritonitis /,peritə'naitis/　　　　　　　腹膜炎
　　peritoneotomy /'peritəuni:əutəmi/　　　　腹腔切开术
　　celiotomy /si:li'ɒtəmi/　　　　　　　　剖腹手术，开腹术
13.　herni(o)　　　　　　　　　　　　　　疝，突出
　　hernioplasty /'hɜ:niəplæsti/　　　　　　疝根治手术
　　herniorrhaphy /hɜ:ni'ɔ:rəfi/　　　　　　疝缝术，疝修补术
14.　appendic(o)　　　　　　　　　　　　阑尾
　　appendicitis /ə,pendi'saitis/　　　　　　阑尾炎，盲肠炎
　　appendicolysis /əpendi'kɒlisis/　　　　　阑尾粘连分离术
15.　ile(o)　　　　　　　　　　　　　　　回肠
　　ileocolitis /iliəukə'laitis/　　　　　　　回肠结肠炎
　　ileotomy /ili'ɒtəmi/　　　　　　　　　回肠切开术
16.　jejun(o)　　　　　　　　　　　　　　空肠
　　jejunitis /dʒi:dʒu'naitis/　　　　　　　空肠炎
　　jejunostomy /dʒidʒu:'nɒstəmi/　　　　　空肠造口术
17.　stomat(o)　　　　　　　　　　　　　口腔
　　stomatitis /,stəumə'taitis/　　　　　　　口腔炎
　　stomatology /,stəumə'tɒlədʒi/　　　　　口腔学
18.　ventr(o)　　　　　　　　　　　　　　腹部，腹，前侧
　　ventrotomy /ven'trɒtəmi/　　　　　　　剖腹术

笔记

ventrodorsal /ventrəʊˈdɔːsəl/　　　　　　　腹背的

ventromedial /ventrəʊˈmiːdiəl/　　　　　　腹正中的

Part Ⅵ　Exercise

Directions: *In this section, only one of the following options is correct, please choose.*

（王蕊蕊　吕小君）

ER-5-32
扫一扫 看一
看

笔 记

Unit 6
Hematology, Immunology and Endocrine Department

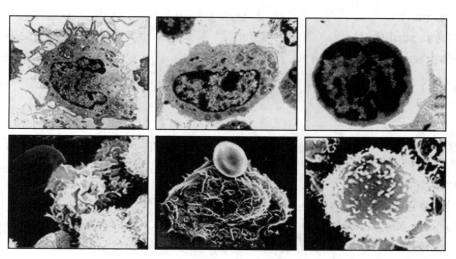

Fig. 6-1   hematology and immunology

Diseases of the soul are more dangerous than those of the body.

心灵上的疾病比身体上的疾病更危险。

——M. T Cicero（西塞罗 .M.T.）

Learning Objectives

Skill focus

1. *Master the symptoms and diagnosis of the patient with disease of immune system.*
2. *Know how to take care of the patient with disease of immune system.*
3. *Understand the diabetes and AIDS.*

Language focus

1. *Have ability of communicating with the patients with disease of immune system.*
2. *Have ability of creating and guessing a new word using roots and prefix or suffix.*

Part I   Listening

This section is designed to test your ability to understand spoken English in nursing or medical contexts. You will hear a selection of recorded materials and you must answer the questions that accompany them. There are TWO parts in this section, Part A and Part B.

ER-6-1
扫一扫 读一读

ER-6-2
扫一扫 看一看

笔记

Part A

Words in Focus

allergy /ˈælədʒi/	n.	过敏性反应
currently /ˈkɜːrəntli/	adv.	当前，目前
pollen /ˈpɑːlən/	n.	花粉；<虫>粉面
antihistamine /ˌænti'histəmin/	n.	抗组织胺药
desensitization /ˌdiːˌsensitaɪˈzeiʃn/	n.	脱敏；脱敏作用
sensitive /ˈsɛnsitiv/	adj.	敏感的；感觉的
susceptible /səˈsɛptibəl/	adj.	易受影响的；易受感染的

Useful Expressions

be aware of	知道；意识到
pay attention to	注意

Text

ER-6-3
扫一扫 听一听

ER-6-4
扫一扫 知情节

Directions: *In this section you will hear a short passage, at the end of the passage, one or more questions will be asked about what was said, decide which the best answer is.*

Background:

　　Mr. Smith doesn't feel well, so he goes to see a doctor. Mr. Smith is diagnosed with allergy. The doctor asks him to conduct an allergy testing to find out what Mr. Smith has an allergy to. The report shows that he has an allergy to pollen. Then the doctor gives him some advice about the ways to avoid allergens.

Comprehension of the text

1. What does Mr. Smith have an allergy to?
   A. pollen　　　　　　　　B. cat　　　　　　　　C. smoke

2. What medicine does the doctor advise Mr. Smith to take?
   A. antihistamine pills and vitamin B
   B. antihistamine pills and vitamin C
   C. sleeping pills and vitamin C

3. According to the conversation, which of the following statements is true?
   A. Good living habits doesn't help to reduce the symptoms.
   B. Mr. Smith should keep the doors and windows open when pollen is high.
   C. Hay fever is no cure for at present.

ER-6-5
扫一扫 读一读

4. Can desensitization course cure the allergy?
   A. Yes　　　　　　　　B. No　　　　　　　　C. Not mentioned

5. According to the doctor's advice, Mr. Smith shouldn't eat _____.
   A. apple　　　　　　　B. bread　　　　　　　C. fish

Part B

ER-6-6
扫一扫 看一看

Words in Focus

immune /ɪˈmjuːn/	adj.	免疫的；有免疫力的
microorganism /ˌmaikroˈɔrgəˌnizəm/	n.	微生物
vital /ˈvaitl/	adj.	至关重要的
utilize /ˈjutilˌaiz/	v.	利用，使用

笔记

inflammatory /in'flæmətɔːri/	adj.	炎性的，发炎的
swell /swɛl/	v.	肿胀
redden /'rɛdn/	v.	（使）变红
overreact /ˌoʊvəri'ækt/	v.	反应过火

Useful Expressions

defend against	保护……不受……，防御
infectious agent	病原体
prevent from	阻止，防止

Text

Directions: *In this section you will hear a short passage, at the end of the passage, one or more questions will be asked about what was said, decide which the best answer is.*

Background:

The immune system is responsible for keeping body healthy free from illness and infections. When the body's immune system does not function properly, it will be disordered and result in disease, including autoimmune diseases, inflammatory diseases and cancer.

Comprehension of the text

1. The immune system protects people from _____.

   A. cells   B. lymph nodes   C. germs and microorganisms

2. How many strategies does our immune system utilize?

   A. two   B. three   C. four

3. An inflammatory reaction can make the body become _____.

   A. warm   B. cold   C. painful

4. The second line of defense is _____.

   A. bloodstream and inflammatory response

   B. skin and gastrointestinal tract

   C. spleen, liver, and lymph nodes

5. Which of the following statements is true?

   A. Peanuts are dangerous to the body.

   B. Inflammatory response can damage tissues and cells.

   C. It is recommended not to treat a high fever.

ER-6-7
扫一扫 听一
听

ER-6-8
扫一扫 知情
节

Part II Speaking

This section is designed to test your speaking ability. After learning the following conversation A and B you will have the ability of speaking skill in medical and nursing working and try to do the following speaking tasks.

Conversation 1

Diabetes

Mr. Green has been in hospital for treatment of diabetes, but he doesn't feel well. The nurse asks him to follow the special diabetic food schedule and do some exercise to control his blood sugar. The nurse reminds him of some side effects of the medicine.

ER-6-9
扫一扫 听一
听

ER-6-10
扫一扫 知情
节

笔记

Jenny:	Good morning. Mr. Green.
Mr. Green:	Good morning. Jenny.
Jenny:	How are you today?
Mr. Green:	I still feel hungry and have a dry throat.
Jenny:	What did you have for your breakfast?
Mr. Green:	I had milk and bread.
Jenny:	For diabetic patients, you know, meals should be frequent but small in quantity.
Mr. Green:	Yes, I know. I just eat a little for my breakfast.
Jenny:	Mr. Green, as the doctor told you, you are diagnosed with type 2 diabetes and you should keep your blood sugar under control by following the specially designed diabetic food schedule.
Mr. Green:	How can I keep a good diet?
Jenny:	Eat plenty of vegetables as they are naturally low in fat and high in fiber. Fat and sugar intake should be limited.
Mr. Green:	Thanks for your advice. I'm sure I can do it.
Jenny:	By the way, regular exercise may help you control your blood sugar. Being overweight and lack of exercise are two main reasons that people fail to control blood sugar.
Mr. Green:	I like doing exercise.
Jenny:	Too much exercise is not allowed. You may bring some cookies in the pocket to avoid the hypoglycemia syndrome while doing exercise.
Mr. Green:	OK, I'll keep that in mind.
Jenny:	Since you've had breakfast, it's time you took medicine.
Mr. Green:	What's it?
Jenny:	It's acarbose which helps to decrease current blood glucose levels.
Mr. Green:	How many do I take?
Jenny:	You take two tablets three times a day, but it may cause gastrointestinal side-effects such as flatulence and diarrhea.
Mr. Green:	OK, I will take care.
Jenny:	The call button is here. You may push it if you need help.
Mr. Green:	Thank you for your kindness.
Jenny:	You are welcome.

(295 words)

Words in Focus

diabetic /ˌdaiə'bɛtik/	adj.	糖尿病的
frequent /'frikwənt/	adj.	频繁的，时常发生的
quantity /'kwɑːntiti/	n.	量，数量；数目
diagnose /ˌdaiəg'nouz/	v.	诊断；判断
schedule /'skedʒuːl/	n.	时刻表，清单，目录
glucose /'gluːkous/	n.	葡萄糖，右旋糖
flatulence /'flætʃələns/	n.	胃肠气胀

ER-6-11
扫一扫 读一读

ER-6-12
扫一扫 看一看

笔记

Useful Expressions

hypoglycemia syndrome   低血糖综合征

side-effect   不良反应

I. Free talk

Directions: *Work in pairs and discuss the following questions after learning the recording of Dialogue One.*

1. What should patients with diabetes avoid eating?

_____

_____

2. What should Mr. Green pay attention to while doing exercise?

_____

_____

II. Comprehension of the text

Directions: *According to the following conversation and complete the sentences.*

1. For diabetic patients, meals should be _____.

   A. frequent but small in quantity

   B. as normal

   C. large

2. What did Mr. Green had for his breakfast?

   A. sandwich and milk   B. bread and milk   C. hamburger

3. Why did the nurse advise Mr. Green to take some cookies in the pocket while doing exercise?

   A. to avoid hypertension

   B. to avoid the hyperglycemia syndrome

   C. to avoid the hypoglycemia syndrome

4. Acarbose may cause some side-effects such as _____ and diarrhea.

   A. headache   B. vomiting   C. flatulence

5. According to the conversation, which of the following does not help to control blood sugar of the diabetes？

   A. moderate exercise

   B. fat and sugar intake

   C. vegetables that is low in fat and high in fiber

ER-6-13
扫一扫 答案
"晓"

Conversation 2

Leukemia

    Robert *doesn't feel well, so he goes to see a doctor. The doctor examines him and advises him to have a blood test and a bone marrow examination. The next day, he brings the reports to the doctor and is diagnosed with acute leukemia. Robert is worried about his illness. The doctor suggests that he should be hospitalized.*

Doctor: Sit down, please. What seems to be bothering you?

Robert: I often feel dizzy and fatigued.

Doctor: How long have you been feeling like this?

Robert: About two weeks.

ER-6-14
扫一扫 听一
听

ER-6-15
扫一扫 知情
节

笔记

Doctor: Did you run any fever?

Robert: Yes.

Doctor: Well, let me take your temperature.

Robert: I 'm afraid I've got a temperature.

Doctor: Yes, 37.8℃. Are there any other symptoms besides these?

Robert: Yes, my nose often bleeds.

Doctor: Does it bleed much?

Robert: Not too much.

Doctor: Do you have night sweats?

Robert: Yes, very often.

Doctor: Have you had any chest pain?

Robert: Yes, I have a pain in my chest when pressing it.

Doctor: All right. Let me examine you. Would you mind taking off your coat?

Robert: OK.

Doctor: There are some bruises on your limbs. Are you hurt?

Robert: No, they just occurred spontaneously.

Doctor: You must have a blood test. I'll take your white blood count and give you a bone marrow examination. Here are your laboratory sheets. After picking up the reports, please bring them back to me.

Robert: Thank you very much, doctor.

(The next day, Robert brings the reports to the doctor)

Patent: What's the result, doctor?

Doctor: Not good. Laboratory tests show leukocytosis, thrombocytopenia and anemia.

Robert: Would you tell me what trouble I suffer from, doctor?

Doctor: According to the symptoms and laboratory tests, I'm sure it's acute leukemia. You should be admitted to hospital immediately.

Robert: What am I supposed to do then?

Doctor: Don't worry. We are determined to try our best.

Robert: Which method should I be treated with?

Doctor: I would recommend the chemotherapy. Another assistant therapy is administered as well, including antibiotics and blood transfusion.

Robert: Is there anything I should pay attention to?

Doctor: A good rest is all you need. Your meals should be light and digestible. I'm sure you'll get well soon. Now you can carry out the admission procedures.

Robert: Thanks. See you.

Doctor: See you.

(329 words)

Words in Focus

leukemia /ljuːˈkiːmiə/	*n.*	<医>白血病
fatigued /fəˈtiːgd/	*adj.*	疲乏的
bruise /bruːz/	*n.*	瘀伤，青肿；擦伤，伤痕
spontaneously /spɒnˈteiniəsli/	*adv.*	自然地，自发地
marrow /ˈmærou/	*n.*	骨髓；脊髓
thrombocytopenia /ˌθrɒmbəˌsaitəˈpiːniːə/	*n.*	血小板减少（症）

ER-6-16
扫一扫 读一读

ER-6-17
扫一扫 看一看

笔记

| chemotherapy /ˌkiːmoʊˈθerəpi/ | n. | 化疗 |
| procedure /prəˈsiːdʒə/ | n. | 程序，手续 |

Useful expressions

| suffer from | 患（某种病），受（某种病痛）折磨 |
| be determined to | 决定；下决心；执意 |

I. Free talk

Directions: *Work in pairs and discuss the following questions after learning the Dialogue Two.*

1. How does the man feel?

_____

_____

2. How should a patient with acute leukemia be treated?

_____

_____

3. Can you list some symptoms of acute leukemia?

_____

_____

II. Comprehension of the text

Directions: *According to the conversation and complete the sentences.*

1. Which of the following is not the patient's symptom?

   A. night sweats   B. fever   C. stomachache

2. The laboratory tests of the patient show leukocytosis, thrombocytopenia and _____.

   A. high blood pressure   B. hyperglycemia   C. anemia

3. How do the bruises on the patient's limbs occur?

   A. They occur spontaneously.   B. He is hurt.   C. Not mentioned.

4. The treatments for the patient's illness include _____, antibiotics and blood transfusion.

   A. chemotherapy   B. operation   C. hormonal therapies

5. The doctor suggests that the patient's meal should be _____.

   A. frequent   B. light and digestible   C. large

Part III   Reading

Text A

Diabetes is a metabolic disorder in human body which does not produce or properly uses insulin, a hormone that is required to convert sugar, starches, and other food into energy. This results in high blood sugar. Over time, high blood sugar can damage many body systems. Know more about diabetes in this text.

Pre-reading

1. What is the diabetes?
2. How many types of diabetes mentioned in the text?

ER-6-18
扫一扫 答案
"晓"

ER-6-19
扫一扫 听一
听

ER-6-20
扫一扫 知情
节

笔记

Diabetes

Diabetes is a metabolic disorder which is characterized by high blood sugar (hyperglycemia). Diabetes develops when the body doesn't make enough insulin or is not able to use insulin effectively, or both. As a result, glucose builds up in the blood instead of being absorbed by cells in the body. The body's cells are then starved of energy despite high blood glucose levels. Over time, high blood glucose damages nerves and blood vessels, leading to complications such as heart disease, stroke, kidney disease, blindness and dental disease.

There are two main types of diabetes. Type 1 diabetes (T1B) usually develops in childhood. The patients with Type 1 diabetes require lifelong insulin injections for survival. Type 2 diabetes (T2B) usually develops in adulthood and is related to obesity, lack of physical activity, and unhealthy diets. This is the more common type of diabetes (representing 90% of diabetic cases worldwide) and treatment may involve lifestyle changes and weight loss alone, or oral medications or even insulin injections.

Hyperglycemia causes a wide variety of symptoms. The classical symptoms of thirst, nocturnal polyuria and rapid weight loss are prominent in type 1 diabetes, but are often absent in patients with type 2 diabetes, many of whom are symptomatic or have non-specific complaints such as chronic fatigue and malaise.

The methods of treatment of diabetes are: dietary and life-style modification, oral anti-diabetic drugs and injected therapies. In patients with type 1 diabetes, urgent treatment with insulin is required and prompt referral to a specialist is usually needed. In patients with type 2 diabetes, the therapy involves advice about dietary and lifestyle modification. Oral anti-diabetic drugs are added in those who do not achieve glycemic targets as a result, or who have severe symptomatic hyperglycemia at diagnosis. Besides these treatments of hyperglycemia, other risk factors for complications of diabetes need to be addressed, including treatment of hypertension and advice on giving up smoking. Eating a balanced diet is vital for people who have diabetes, so work with your doctor or dietitian to set up a menu plan. If you have type 1 diabetes, the timing of your insulin dosage is determined by activity and diet. When you eat and how much you eat are just as important as what you eat. Usually, doctors recommend three small meals and three to four snacks every day to maintain the proper balance between sugar and insulin in the blood. Another crucial element in a treatment program for diabetes is exercise. Exercise improves your body's use of insulin and may lower blood sugar levels.

The aims of treatment are to relieve the symptoms of hyperglycemia and to achieve as near normal metabolism as is practicable, while avoiding hypoglycemia and therapeutic side-effects. The nearer the body weight approaches the ideal level and the closer the blood sugar is kept to normal, the more the total metabolic profile is improved and the lower the incidence of vascular disease and of specific diabetic complications.

(491 words)

Words in Focus

disorder /dis'ɔ:də(r)/	*n.*	（身心机能的）失调
hyperglycemia /ˌhaipəglaiˈsi:miə/	*n.*	多糖症，高血糖症
insulin /ˈinsəlin/	*n.*	胰岛素

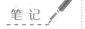
笔记

absorb /əbˈsɔrb/	v.	吸收（液体、气体等）
vessel /ˈvɛsəl/	n.	血管
survival /sərˈvaivl/	n.	幸存，生存
polyuria /ˌpɒliˈjuəriə/	n.	多尿（症）
nocturnal /nɑːkˈtɜːrnl/	adj.	夜的，夜间的
prominent /ˈprɑːminənt/	adj.	突出的，杰出的
dietary /ˈdaiəˌtɛri/	adj.	饮食的，规定食物的
referral /riˈfɜːrəl/	n.	介绍，指引
modification /ˌmɑːdifiˈkeiʃn/	n.	修改，修正
symptomatic /ˌsimtəˈmætik, ˌsimp-/	adj.	有症状的
crucial /ˈkruʃəl/	adj.	极其重要的
vascular /ˈvæskjulə/	adj.	血管的；脉管的

ER-6-21
扫一扫 读一读

ER-6-22
扫一扫 看一看

Useful Expressions

instead of	而不是……
give up	放弃；投降
set up	建立；准备

Post-reading

I. Comprehension of the text

Choose the best answer to complete each sentence with the information from the text.

1. Which of the following is not the cause of the diabetes?

    A. Glucose is absorbed by cells in the body.

    B. The body doesn't make enough insulin.

    C. The body isn't able to use insulin effectively.

2. Which of the following is not the complication of the diabetes?

    A. heart disease　　　　B. stomachache　　　　C. blindness

3. Which of the following is not the symptom of diabetes?

    A. thirst　　　　B. weight loss　　　　C. headache

4. Which of the following can't control the blood sugar of the diabetes?

    A. exercise　　　　B. a balanced diet　　　　C. sleep

5. The time of insulin dosage depends on _____.

    A. activity and diet　　　　B. weight　　　　C. blood sugar level

II. Vocabulary activities

Find a word or phrase from the box below to complete each sentence. Change word forms where necessary.

insulin	absorb	vascular	complication	symptom
hyperglycemia	result in	modification	injection	risk

1. Diabetes is a chronic and potentially life-threatening condition where the body loses its ability to produce _____.

2. The most common diabetes _____ include frequent urination, intense thirst, weight loss and fatigue.

3. Hyperglycemia can cause _____ disease.

4. For Type 1 diabetics there will always be a need for insulin _____ throughout their life.

笔记

85

ER-6-23
扫一扫 答案
"晓"

ER-6-24
扫一扫 练一
练

ER-6-25
扫一扫 听一
听

ER-6-26
扫一扫 知情
节

5. Normally, glucose is _____ by cells.

6. Overweight and obese people have a much higher _____ of developing type 2 diabetes compared to those with a healthy body weight.

7. Type 2 diabetics can control the disease by dietary _____.

8. _____-when blood sugar is too high -has a bad effect on the patient.

9. Diabetes can _____ other serious problems. These problems are known as diabetes complications.

10. Heart disease, stroke, kidney disease, blindness and dental disease are _____ of diabetes.

III. Supplementary

Text B

> AIDS has had a great impact on society, both as an illness and as a source of discrimination. There are many misconceptions about AIDS such as the belief that it can be transmitted by casual non-sexual contact. In this text, we'll learn more about AIDS.
>
> ### Pre-reading
> 1. What is the AIDS short for?
> 2. How many ways is the HIV transmitted?

AIDS

The acquired immune deficiency syndrome (AIDS) is a series of conditions caused by infection with the human immunodeficiency virus (HIV). It may also be referred to as HIV disease or HIV infection. The virus causes an immune deficiency by attacking a type of white blood cell that helps to fight infections. Because this leads to various diseases, not a single illness, AIDS is referred to as a syndrome.

The symptoms of AIDS vary depending on the stage of infection. The initial infection is symptomatic in most cases and usually occurs in the first few weeks after exposure. Many are unaware of their status until later stages. Many individuals develop an influenza-like illness including fever, headache, rash or sore throat, while others have no significant symptoms. As the infection progresses, it interferes more and more with the immune system, making the person much more susceptible to common infections, like tuberculosis, as well as opportunistic infections and tumors that do not usually affect people who have working immune systems. The late symptoms of the infection are referred to as AIDS. This stage is often complicated by an infection of the lung known as pneumocystis pneumonia, severe weight loss, skin lesions caused by Kaposi's sarcoma, or other AIDS-defining conditions.

HIV is present in blood, semen and other body fluids such as breast milk. Exposure to infected fluid leads to a risk of contracting infection, which is dependent on the integrity of the exposed site, the type and volume of body fluid, and the viral load. HIV can enter either as free virus or within cells. HIV is transmitted primarily through unprotected sexual intercourse, contaminated blood transfusions, hypodermic needles, and from mother to child during pregnancy, delivery, or breastfeeding. Some bodily fluids, such as saliva and tears, do not transmit HIV. Individuals cannot become infected through ordinary day-to-day contact such as kissing, hugging, shaking hands, or sharing personal objects, food or water.

笔记

Efforts to prevent the spread of AIDS focus on sex education and the use of condoms. Other measures, such as male circumcision, may also help to cut the risk of sexually transmitted infection.

There is no cure for AIDS, but treatments are available that combat its onset. Antiviral drugs work by slowing the replication of HIV in the body. These drugs need to be used in combination because the virus readily mutates, creating new and often drug-resistant strains. Such treatments are expensive, however, and are still denied to millions of people in the developing world.

In the future, the hope is for an AIDS vaccine that would prevent HIV infection. Researchers are currently working on more than 30 potential candidates.

(438 words)

Words in Focus

acquire /əˈkwaiə/	v.	学到；获得，取得
deficiency /diˈfiʃənsi/	n.	缺乏；缺点，缺陷
interfere /ˌintəˈfiə/	v.	干预，干涉
tumor /ˈtjuːmə/	n.	瘤
semen /ˈsiːmən/	n.	精液
fluid /ˈfluːid/	n.	液体
exposure /ikˈspouʒə(r)/	n.	暴露
integrity /inˈtɛgriti/	n.	完整
contaminate /kənˈtæmiˌneit/	v.	污染
mutate /ˈmjuːteit/	v.	变异
replication /ˌrɛpliˈkeiʃən/	n.	复制
circumcision /ˌsɜːrkəmˈsiʒn/	n.	割礼，包皮环切（术）
lesion /ˈliːʒən/	n.	损害
potential /pəˈtɛnʃəl/	adj.	潜在的，有可能的
candidate /ˈkændiˌdeit, -dit/	n.	候选人

ER-6-27
扫一扫 读一读

Useful Expressions

opportunistic infection	机会性感染
pneumocystis pneumonia	卡氏肺囊虫性肺炎
Kaposi's sarcoma	卡波西肉瘤

ER-6-28
扫一扫 看一看

Post–reading

I. Comprehension of the text

Choose the best answer to complete each sentence with the information from the text.

1. HIV causes an immune deficiency by attacking a type of _____.

    A. white blood cell　　　B. red blood cell　　　C. nerve

2. The symptoms of AIDS is dependent on the _____ of infection.

    A. way　　　B. stage　　　C. time

3. HIV is present in _____, semen and other body fluids such as breast milk.

    A. saliva　　　B. tears　　　C. blood

4. HIV is transmitted through unprotected sexual intercourse, _____, hypodermic needles, and from mother to child during pregnancy, delivery, or breastfeeding.

笔记

A. contaminated blood transfusions

B. kissing

C. hugging

5. Antiviral drugs work by _____ the replication of HIV in the body.

    A. increasing   B. stopping   C. slowing

II. Vocabulary activities

Find a word or phrase from the box below to complete each sentence. There are more words and phrases than you need to fill in all the sentences. Change word forms where necessary.

depend on	infect	locate	condition	transmit	prevent
as well as	as a result	delivery	deny	ordinary	lead to

ER-6-29
扫一扫 答案
"晓"

1. An ordinary cold can soon _____ a fever.

2. I strongly suspect that most _____ people would agree with me.

3. Vitamin C is supposed to _____ colds.

4. The mother had an easy _____.

5. A single mosquito can _____ a large number of people.

6. They all _____ ever having seen her.

7. Some diseases are _____ from one generation to the next.

8. Whether the game will be played _____ the weather.

ER-6-30
扫一扫 练一
练

9. The government has encouraged its people to better their _____.

10. Flowers are chosen for their scent _____ their look.

III. Supplementary

Part Ⅳ   Writing

Writing a Medical Certificate

Instructions:

    This article is about documentation relating to a medical examination. A medical certificate (sometimes referred to as a doctor's certificate) is a statement from a physician or other health care provider that attests to the result of a medical examination of a patient. It can serve as a "sick note" (documentation that an employee is unfit for work) or evidence of a health condition. Medical certificates are sometimes required to obtain certain health benefits from an employer, make an insurance claim, for tax purposes, or for certain legal procedures. Medical certificates are used to indicate eligibility of activity, such as the use of disabled parking. Medical certificates can also be used to describe a medical condition a person has, such as blindness. Medical certificates are often used to certify that someone is free of contagious diseases, drug addiction, mental illness, or other health issues.

Sentence Patterns:

    中文证明书常以"兹证明……"开始,英语多译为:

    This is to certify that...

    I have the pleasure in certifying that...

笔 记

I hereby certify that...

It's my pleasure to give evidence that...

A certificatre usually consists of the following parts:

1. **the heading** (certificate)
2. **the body** (the main content of the certificate)
3. **the signature** (handwritten or typed)

Examples:

Certificate of Admission

The People's Hospital of Chizhou

This is to certify that Zhang Jun, male, aged 36, has a high fever of 39.2℃ and a very bad sore throat. He was admitted to our hospital for medical treatment on December 12th, 2015 and is not be able to return to work for about four days.

Signature

The People's Hospital of Chizhou (seal)

Practice:

兹证明病人李军，男，42 岁，因患腹膜炎（peritonitis）于 2015 年 12 月 15 日住院。经立即施行手术和 7 天治疗后，现已痊愈，将于 2015 年 12 月 22 日出院。建议在家休息一个星期后再上班工作。

ER-6-31
扫一扫 答案
"晓"

Part Ⅴ   Enriching your word power

1.	chrom(o)-	色
	chromometer /krə'mɒmitə/	比色计
	chromatosome /k'rəʊmitəzəm/ 同 chromosome	染色体
2.	immun(o)-	免疫
	immunochemistry /ˌimjuːnəʊ'kemistri/	免疫化学
	immunotherapy /i'mjuːnəʊ'θerəpi/	免疫疗法
3.	lymph(o)-	淋巴
	lymphocyte /'limfəsait/	淋巴球，淋巴细胞
	lymphocytoma /limfəsai'təmə/	淋巴瘤
4.	hemat(o)-; hem(o)-	血
	hematocyte /'hemətəʊsait/ 同 hemocyte	血细胞
	hemoglobin /ˌhiːməʊ'gləʊbin/	血红蛋白
5.	Emia-	血症
	hypercalcemia /haipəkæl'siːmiə/	血钙过多
	hyperazotemia /haipərəzəʊ'tiːmiə/	高氮血症

笔记

6.　erythr(o)-　　　　　　　　　　　　　　　　　红
　　erythroblast /ɪ'riθrəblæst/　　　　　　　　　成红血球细胞
　　erythrocyturia /əriθrə'situːriə/ 同 hematuria　血尿

7.　leuk(o)-　　　　　　　　　　　　　　　　　白
　　leukocyte /'ljuːkəu,sait/　　　　　　　　　　白细胞，白血球
　　leukorrhea /,ljuːkəu'riːə/　　　　　　　　　白带

8.　cyt(o)-　　　　　　　　　　　　　　　　　　细胞
　　cytobiology /saitəubai'ɒlədʒi/　　　　　　　细胞生物学
　　cytopenia /,saitə'piːniə/　　　　　　　　　　血细胞减少

9.　macro-　　　　　　　　　　　　　　　　　　大，长，巨
　　macrogenesy /'mækrədʒiːnisi/ 同 gigantism　巨人症
　　macrophagocyte /məkrə'fægəsait/　　　　　巨噬细胞

10.　micro-　　　　　　　　　　　　　　　　　小，微，细
　　microbe /'maikrəub/　　　　　　　　　　　微生物，细菌
　　microangiopathy 'maikrəuændʒi'ɒpəθi/　　微血管病

11.　thromb(o)-　　　　　　　　　　　　　　　血栓
　　thromboangiitis /θrɒmbəuændʒi'aitis/　　　血栓（性）脉管炎
　　thrombosis /θrɒm'bəusis/　　　　　　　　血栓形成
　　thrombocyte /'θrɒmbəsait/　　　　　　　小板，凝血细胞

12.　crin(o)-　　　　　　　　　　　　　　　　分泌
　　endocrine /'endəukrin/　　　　　　　　　内分泌
　　crinophagy /krinə'fædʒi/　　　　　　　　胞内分泌吞噬

13.　end(o)-　　　　　　　　　　　　　　　　在内部
　　endocrine /'endəukrin/　　　　　　　　　内分泌

14.　varic(o)-　　　　　　　　　　　　　　　静脉曲张
　　varicosis /væri'kəusis/　　　　　　　　　静脉曲张病
　　varicophlebitis /værikəfli'baitis/　　　　曲张静脉炎

15.　aden(o)-　　　　　　　　　　　　　　　腺
　　adenocarcinoma /,ædnəu,kɑːsə'nəumə/　腺癌
　　adenoma /,ædə'nəumə/　　　　　　　　腺瘤

16.　thym(o)-　　　　　　　　　　　　　　　胸腺
　　thymoma /θai'məumə/　　　　　　　　　胸腺瘤
　　thymosin /'θaiməsɪn/　　　　　　　　　胸腺素

17.　hormon(o)-　　　　　　　　　　　　　　激素
　　hormonosis /hɔːmɒ'nəusis/　　　　　　　激素过多症
　　hormonotherapy /hɔːmɒnəu'θerəpi/　　　激素疗法

18.　thyr(o); thyroid(o)-　　　　　　　　　　甲状腺
　　hyperthyroidism /,haipə'θairɔidizəm/　　　甲状腺机能亢进
　　thyroxine /θai'rɒksi(ː)n/　　　　　　　　甲状腺素

19.　adren(o)-; adrenal(o)-　　　　　　　　　肾上腺
　　adrenocortical /ə,driːnəu'kɔːtikəl/　　　　肾上腺皮质的
　　adrenotrophin /ædre'nɒtrəfin/　　　　　促皮质素，促肾上腺皮质激素

20.　ket(o)-; keton-　　　　　　　　　　　　酮基

笔记

ketoacidosis /kiːtəʊæsiˈdəʊsis/　　　　　　酮酸中毒
ketonuria /kiːtəʊˈnjʊəriə/　　　　　　　　酮尿

Part Ⅵ　Exercise

Directions: *In this section, only one of the following options is correct, please choose.*

（陈精华　吕小君）

ER-6-32
扫一扫 看一看

笔记

Unit 7
Department of Neurology

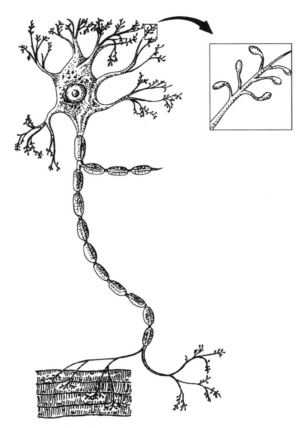

Fig. 7-1 department of neurology

Early to bed and early to rise, makes a man healthy, wealthy and wise.

早睡早起会使人健康、富有和聪明。

——（Benjamin Franklin 富兰克林）

Learning Objectives

Skill focus

1. *Be able to perform pre-procedure and post-procedure interventions related to neurologic diagnostic tests.*

2. *Be able to perform the basic nursing interventions related to meningitis and seizures.*

3. *Be able to perform the basic nursing interventions related to Parkinson's disease and stroke.*

Language focus

1. *Be able to use the words, phrases related to Neurological nursing.*

笔记

2. *Be able to tell nursing instructions related to Neurological nursing.*

3. *Be able to write a nursing assessment.*

Part Ⅰ　Listening

This section is designed to test your ability to understand spoken English in nursing or medical contexts. You will hear a selection of recorded materials and you must answer the questions that accompany them. There are TWO parts in this section, Part A and Part B.

Part A

Words in Focus

diagnostic /ˌdaiəɡˈnɑːstik/	*adj.*	诊断的，判断的
multiple /ˈmʌltipəl/	*adj.*	多重的，多个的，复杂的
denture /ˈdɛntʃ ə/	*n.*	（一副）假牙，托牙
hairpin /ˈheəpin/	*n.*	发夹
underwire /ˈʌndə wair/	*n.*	胸罩的钢丝
radiologist /ˌreidiˈɑːlədʒist/	*n.*	放射线技师
analyze /ˈænəˌlaiz/	*vt.*	分析，分解，解释
refer /riˈfə/	*v.*	提到，针对，归因于……

ER-7-1
扫一扫 读一读

ER-7-2
扫一扫 看一看

Useful Expressions

CT scan	分层造影扫描，CT 扫描
medical test	医学检查
X-rays	X 射线
loose-fitting	宽松而合体
prior to	在……之前

Text

Directions: *In this section you will hear a short passage. At the end of the passage, 5 questions will be asked about what you have heard, choose the best answer for each question.*

Background:

　　Sophie, a girl, will take a CT scan ordered by her doctor, and she is talking something about it with the nurse-in-charge.

Comprehension of the text

1. Comparing with traditional X-rays, CT scan images are _____.

　　A. more detailed　　　　B. less detailed　　　　C. equally detailed

2. Metal objects need to be removed _____.

　　A. before the test　　　　B. after the test　　　　C. during the test

3. According to the passage, which of the following statements is true?

　　A. Sophie does not have to remove her bra whether or not containing metal underwire.

　　B. Sophie does not have to remove her bra containing metal underwire.

　　C. Sophie must remove her bra containing metal underwire.

4. What will the patient feel during the test?

ER-7-3
扫一扫 听一听

ER-7-4
扫一扫 知情节

笔记

A. She will not feel uncomfortable.

B. She will feel rather uncomfortable.

C. Not mentioned.

5. Who will offer CT scan result?

A. Physician who referred you for the exam.

B. A radiologist.

C. Both A and B.

Part B

Words in Focus

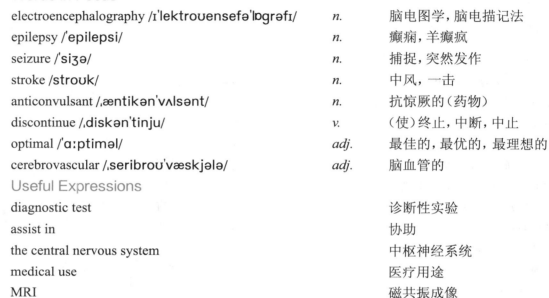

electroencephalography /ɪˈlektroʊensefəˈlɒgrəfɪ/	*n.*	脑电图学,脑电描记法
epilepsy /ˈepilepsi/	*n.*	癫痫,羊癫疯
seizure /ˈsiʒə/	*n.*	捕捉,突然发作
stroke /stroʊk/	*n.*	中风,一击
anticonvulsant /ˌæntikənˈvʌlsənt/	*n.*	抗惊厥的（药物）
discontinue /ˌdiskənˈtinju/	*v.*	（使）终止,中断,中止
optimal /ˈɑːptiməl/	*adj.*	最佳的,最优的,最理想的
cerebrovascular /ˌseribroʊˈvæskjələ/	*adj.*	脑血管的

Useful Expressions

diagnostic test	诊断性实验
assist in	协助
the central nervous system	中枢神经系统
medical use	医疗用途
MRI	磁共振成像

Text

Directions: *You're going to hear a conversation. listen to it carefully, then fill in the missing words and choose the right answer to each question.*

Background:

　　The head nurse of Neurological Department and nurse students are talking about some diagnostic tests.

Comprehension of the text

1. EEG can be used to detect the following conditions except _____.

A. epilepsy　　　　　　B. stroke　　　　　　C. meningitis

2. Before taking EEG, the patient shouldn't take anticonvulsant. _____

A. yes　　　　　　　　B. no　　　　　　　　C. not mentioned

3. Comparing with CT scan, MRI is _____.

A. better visualized　　B. more commonly used　　C. more sensitive

4. MRI is used to detected the following medical conditions EXCEPT _____.

A. neurological cancers　　B. cerebrovascular disease　　C. pelvic inflammation

5. The patient should remove metal items and electronic devices when taking MRI examination _____.

A. yes　　　　　　　　B. no　　　　　　　　C. not mentioned

ER-7-5
扫一扫 读一读

ER-7-6
扫一扫 看一看

ER-7-7
扫一扫 听一听

ER-7-8
扫一扫 知情节

笔记

Part Ⅱ　Speaking

This section is designed to test your speaking ability. After learning the following conversation A and B you will have some abilities of speaking skill in medical and nursing working context. Try to do the following speaking tasks.

Conversation 1

At the Consulting Room

Mr. Brown, a 28-year-old clerk, began to have a severe headache 2 days ago, he became less active than before. He often feels sleepy and tired and difficult to flex his neck. So he decides to see a doctor.

ER-7-9
扫一扫 听一听

ER-7-10
扫一扫 知情节

Doctor:	Good morning, Mr. Brown. I am Dr. Smith. Do you mind if I use a tape recorder so I don't have to take notes?
Mr. Brown:	Of course not.
Doctor:	Mr. Brown, what do you think is wrong with you?
Mr. Brown:	Well, recently, I feel rigid to move my head, and it aches terribly. I often feel sleepy and tired.
Doctor:	I see, when did the pain begin?
Mr. Brown:	About 2 days ago.
Doctor:	Could you describe it?
Mr. Brown:	It's a sharp pain, just like something pricks my brain.
Doctor:	How long will it last?
Mr. Brown:	It lasts all day long, and it's killing me.
Doctor:	You mean the pain kills you?
Mr. Brown:	Sorry, I really want to say that it is a terrible pain.
Doctor:	Do you feel anything else wrong when the pain comes?
Mr. Brown:	I feel sick and want to throw up.
Doctor:	I see, please lie down, and I will examine you. How long have you had these rashes?
Mr. Brown:	About 3 days.
Doctor:	And tell me when you felt difficult to bend you neck.
Mr. Brown:	It came with the headache.
Doctor:	Did you suffer from any disease recently?
Mr. Brown:	I caught a cold two weeks ago, but it's over. what's wrong with me?
Doctor:	It seems like a meningitis.
Mr. Brown:	Is it serious?
Doctor:	Take it easy, it is a kind of inflammation caused by bacterial and viral organisms. Upper respiratory infections may cause it.
Mr. Brown:	I get it.
Doctor:	I'll ask the nurse to give you an injection to relieve your pain.
Mr. Brown:	Thank you.
Doctor:	And you should be admitted to the hospital.

笔记

Mr. Brown:	May I take some medicine or treat it at a clinic? You know, I'm quite busy.
Doctor:	You know, you need further examinations and tests to confirm it, and if it is meningitis, some precautions must be taken.
Mr. Brown:	Would you please tell me something about them?
Doctor:	Well, your vital signs and ICP must be monitored.
Mr. Brown:	What is ICP?
Doctor:	It is intracranial pressure, a measure to tell the pressure in your brain, when it is higher than usual you will feel headache. and it would be fatal if it becomes extremely high.
Mr. Brown:	I see.
Doctor:	And once the meningitis is diagnosed, some isolation precautions will be necessary.
Mr. Brown:	In that case, I will follow your advice.
Doctor:	And the head of your bed must be elevated to 30 degrees, you should avoid neck flexion, and no visitors are permitted.
Mr. Brown:	Thanks a lot, doctor.
Doctor:	Miss Wilson will accompany you to Neurological Department. Shall I call your family to prepare something for you?
Mr. Brown:	All right, I'd much appreciate for your help.

(519 words)

ER-7-11
扫一扫 读一读

ER-7-12
扫一扫 看一看

Words in Focus

rigid /ˈridʒid/	*adj.*	僵硬的；严格的
prick /prik/	*vt.*	刺，扎
rash /ræʃ/	*n.*	（皮）疹；爆发
meningitis /ˌmɛninˈdʒaitis/	*n.*	脑膜炎
bacterial /bækˈtiəriəl/	*adj.*	细菌的；细菌性的
viral /ˈvairəl/	*adj.*	病毒的，病毒引起的
organism /ˈɔːgənizəm/	*n.*	有机体；生物体；微生物
precaution /priˈkɔʃən/	*n.*	预防措施；预防
hospitalization /ˌhɒspitəlaiˈzeiʃən/	*n.*	住院治疗；送入医院
neurological /ˌnuərəˈlɑːdʒikl/	*adj.*	神经学的；神经病学的

Useful Expressions

throw up	呕吐
upper respiratory infection	上呼吸道感染
isolation precaution	隔离措施
intracranial pressure(ICP)	颅内压

I. Free talk

Directions: *Work in pairs and discuss the following questions after listening to Dialogue One.*

1. Explain to your partner the methods of interviews of pain.

_____

_____

_____

笔记

2. What is wrong with Mr. Brown?

_____

_____

_____

II. Comprehension of the text

Directions: Complete the sentences according to the conversation.

1. Headache, _____ and rigid of neck are all signs and symptoms meningitis.

    A. rashes   B. dizzy   C. sick

2. When taking care of patients suffering from meningitis, the following steps are necessary except _____.

    A. vital signs and ICP must be monitored

    B. some isolation precautions will be necessary

    C. the patient can be treated in the clinics

3. Which one of the following statements about ICP is not correct? _____

    A. ICP indicates the pressure in one's brain.

    B. The headache will occur when ICP is higher than usual.

    C. The increase of ICP is the typical sign of meningitis.

4. The nursing procedures of meningitis include the following steps EXCEPT _____.

    A. the head of patient's bed must be elevated to 30 degrees.

    B. no visitors are permitted to visit the patient during hospitalization.

    C. the patient can move his or her head whenever he or she wants.

5. Meningitis may be caused by which of the following reasons? _____

    A. Upper respiratory infections

    B. Hypertension

    C. Stroke

ER-7-13
扫一扫 答案
"晓"

ER-7-14
扫一扫 听一
听

ER-7-15
扫一扫 知情
节

Conversation 2

Seizures

Tommy Johns is a 5 years old boy. He is clever and lovely. Just now, he told his mother that he felt something wrong and scared about that, then became tonic-clonic and lost his consciousness. Not knowing what to do, Mrs. Johns called their community nurse for help.

Nurse:	Hello, this is Julia George, the community nurse, what can I do for you?
Mrs. Johns:	Hello, nurse, this is Mrs. Johns speaking, a seizure attack happens to my son, I don't know what to do.
Nurse:	Don't be nervous, is this the first attack?
Mrs. Johns:	No, it happened to him 3 week ago.
Nurse:	I get it, Mrs. Johns, do what I tell you, ease him down to the ground, let the seizure develop, do not try to stop or disturb it, place him in a side-lying position.
Mrs. Johns:	Yes, that's done.
Nurse:	Put a pillow or something soft under his head, and keep everything away from his mouth and nose, unfasten his cloth, let him breathe easily.
Mrs. Johns:	OK. Oh, my god, he is vomiting.

笔记

97

Nurse:	Turn him to one side, and do not place anything in his mouth or give him any liquid to drink.
Mrs. Johns:	All right. Now he looks less rigid than before.
Nurse:	How long does this last?
Mrs. Johns:	About 20 seconds.
Nurse:	Mrs. Johns, is there anybody else with you ?
Mrs. Johns:	Yes, his father is staying with him now.
Nurse:	Good, Mrs. Johns, tell me something about you son's seizures, please.
Mrs. Johns:	Yes, he caught a bad cold 6 weeks ago, when he recovered and just before being discharged from hospital, the first attack came, his doctor told me that seizures attack might happen to him again, and this is the first attack happened at home. Oh, the seizure comes again.
Nurse:	Keep doing what I told you just now.
Mrs. Johns:	It's gone.
Nurse:	Generally, the seizure's off and on may last about 1 minute.
Mrs. Johns:	You are right, it's over. it seems that he is sleeping.
Nurse:	Now, please remove him to bed, make sure there is no any hazards or hard objects around him, and keep at least one of you staying with the child until he fully recovers.
Mrs. Johns:	All right. And what should I do next?
Nurse:	Mrs. Johns, please write down his seizures attack time, duration, things accompany it. By the way, did you notice anything different just before it?
Mrs. Johns:	Just now, we were having breakfast, Tommy told me that he felt hot in his stomach, and scared, then he stood up and tried to hold his father and the attack caught him, luckily, my husband hold him.
Nurse:	Did he take any kind of medicine?
Mrs. Johns:	Yes, his doctor has prescribed some medicines for him.
Nurse:	OK, be sure to let Tommy take them on time, and you should do some seizure precautions.
Mrs. Johns:	All right, what should I do?
Nurse:	Remember to raise the side rails when he is sleeping or resting, and pad the side rails and other hard objects.
Mrs. Johns:	You are right, and he must wear a protective helmet and padding during activities like bicycle riding, skateboarding, is that right?.
Nurse:	Exactly. and call me again when necessary.
Mrs. Johns:	Thank you very much.

(559 words)

Words in Focus

unfasten /ʌnˈfæsən/	vt.	松开，解开
discharge /disˈtʃɑːdʒ/	vi.	（病人）出院
hazard /ˈhæzəd/	n.	危险，冒险的事
pad /pæd/	vt.	给……装衬垫
helmet /ˈhɛlmit/	n.	头盔，钢盔

ER-7-16
扫一扫 读一读

笔记

Useful Expressions

side-lying position   侧卧位

off and on   断断续续地

I. Free talk

Directions: Work in pairs and discuss the following questions after listening to Dialogue Two.

1. What did the woman call for?

    _____

    _____

    _____

2. Why is the patient put in the side-lying position?

    _____

    _____

    _____

3. If you are a nurse to care a patient undergoing seizures, what should you do first?

    _____

    _____

    _____

II. Comprehension of the text

Directions: Complete the sentences according to the conversation.

1. Seizures can be caused by _____, toxicity, circulatory or metabolic disorders.

    A. angry   B. depression   C. infection

2. The procedures tackling with seizures attack are the following ones except _____.

    A. Place him in a side-lying position

    B. Ease him down to the ground

    C. Stop the client's limbs from trembling

3. How to keep the patient safe when seizures attack happens? _____

    A. Remove him or her to bed.

    B. Place a pillow or something soft under his head.

    C. Give him or her some liquid.

4. When the seizures attack is over and the patient falls into sleep, which one of the following steps is proper for the patient? _____

    A. Remove him or her to bed from the ground.

    B. Wear a protective helmet for him or her.

    C. Place something in his mouth in case of vomiting.

5. Which of the following precautions is not correct to a patient suffering from seizures?

    _____

    A. Raise the side rails when he or she is sleeping or resting.

    B. Pad the side rails and other hard objects.

    C. Ask him or her to keep in a side-lying position when sleeping or resting.

ER-7-17
扫一扫 看一
看

ER-7-18
扫一扫 答案
"晓"

笔 记

Part Ⅲ   Reading

Text A

ER-7-19
扫一扫 听一听

ER-7-20
扫一扫 知情节

> Stroke, one of the most commonly suffered diseases nowadays, has drown so many medical staff's attention to its causes, signs and symptoms, assessment and interventions.
>
> ***Pre-reading***
>
> 1. What is stroke?
> 2. What's the reason of stroke?
> 3. How to cope with acute phrase of stroke?

Stroke (brain attack)

Stroke, also known as cerebrovascular accident (CVA), cerebrovascular insult (CVI), or brain attack, is when poor blood flow to the brain results in cell death. There are two main types of stroke: ischemic, due to lack of blood flow, and hemorrhagic, due to bleeding. They result in part of the brain not functioning properly.

Signs and symptoms of a stroke may include inability to move or feel on one side of the body, problems of understanding or speaking, feeling like the world is spinning, or loss of vision to one side among others. Signs and symptoms often appear soon after the stroke has occurred. Hemorrhagic strokes may also be associated with a severe headache.

The main risk factor for stroke is high blood pressure. Other risk factors include tobacco smoking, obesity, high blood cholesterol, diabetes mellitus, previous TIA, and atrial fibrillation among others. An ischemic stroke is typically caused by blockage of a blood vessel. A hemorrhagic stroke is caused by bleeding either directly into the brain or into the space surrounding the brain. Bleeding may occur due to a brain aneurysm. Diagnosis is typically with medical imaging such as a CT scan or MRI scan along with a physical exam. Other tests such as an electrocardiogram (ECG) and blood tests are done to determine risk factors and rule out other possible causes. Low blood sugar may cause similar symptoms.

Disability affects 75% of stroke survivors enough to decrease their employ ability. Stroke can affect people physically, mentally, emotionally, or a combination of the three. The results of stroke vary widely depending on size and location of the lesion. Dysfunction corresponds to areas in the brain that have been damaged.

Treatment of stroke varies according to the underlying cause of the stroke, thromboembolic (ischemic) or hemorrhagic. Definitive therapy of ischemic stroke is aimed at removing the blockage by breaking the clot down (thrombolysis), or by removing it mechanically (thrombectomy). Thrombectomy may improve outcomes if done early in those with an anterior circulation large artery clot. People with intracerebral hemorrhage require neurosurgical evaluation to detect and treat the cause of the bleeding, although many may not need surgery.

Good nursing care is fundamental in maintaining skin care, feeding, hydration, positioning, and monitoring vital signs. During the acute phase of stroke, maintaining a patent airway and administer oxygen as prescribed is necessary. While in the post-acute phase, the gag reflex and

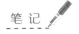

笔记

ability to swallow must be assessed before providing sips of fluids

(445 words)

Words in Focus

ischemic /isˈkiːmik/	*adj.*	缺血性的
hemorrhagic /ˈhemərædʒik/	*adj.*	出血性的
atrial /ˈeitriəl/	*adj.*	心房的
fibrillation /ˌfaibrəˈleiʃən/	*n.*	肌纤维震颤
aneurysm /ˈænjəˌrizəm/	*n.*	动脉瘤
disability /ˌdisəˈbiliti/	*n.*	残疾，无力
thromboembolic /ˌθrɒmbəˈembəlik/	*adj.*	血栓栓子的
thrombolysis /θˈrɒmbɒlisis/	*n.*	溶栓
thrombectomy /θrɒmˈbektəmi/	*n.*	血栓切除术
anterior /ænˈtiəriə/	*adj.*	位于前部的
intracerebral /ˌintrəsiˈriːbrəl/	*adj.*	大脑内的
patent /ˈpætnt/	*adj.*	专利的，明摆着的

ER-7-21
扫一扫 读一读

ER-7-22
扫一扫 看一看

Useful Expressions

cerebrovascular accident	脑血管意外
be associated with	和…联系在一起，与…有关
high blood pressure	高血压
high blood cholesterol	高胆固醇
atrial fibrillation	心房颤动
brain aneurysm	脑动脉瘤
gag reflex	呕吐反射

Post-reading

I. Comprehension of text

Ⅰ) **Choose the best answer to complete each sentence with the information from the text.**

1. When poor blood flows to the brain, the results of cell death and _____ may occur.

    A. high blood cholesterol　　B. improper brain function　　C. diabetes mellitus

2. Signs and symptoms of a stroke may include the following aspects except _____.

    A. an inability to move or feel on one side of the body

    B. feeling like the world is spinning

    C. low blood sugar

3. The main risk factor of stroke is _____.

    A. tobacco smoking　　B. high blood pressure　　C. high blood cholesterol

4. Treatment of ischemic stroke is removing the blockage, it may include thrombolysis and _____.

    A. removing it mechanically　　B. surgery　　C. medication

5. During the acute phase of stroke, it is necessary to maintain a patent airway and _____ when caring for the patients.

    A. administer oxygen as prescribed

    B. provide sips of fluids

    C. detect and treat the cause of stroke

笔记

Ⅱ) **Read the following statements and then decide whether they are true or false based on the information from the text. Write T for truth and F for false in the space provided.**

_____ 1. Poor blood flow to the brain may result in the brain not functioning properly.

_____ 2. Signs and symptoms of stroke always appear soon after the stroke has occurred.

_____ 3. Low blood sugar may cause the feeling like the world is spinning.

_____ 4. Treatment of stroke varies according to the reasons of the stroke.

_____ 5. While in the post-acute phase of the stroke, maintaining a patent airway and administer oxygen as prescribed are necessary.

II. Vocabulary activities

Find a word or phrase from the box below to complete each sentence. Change word forms where necessary.

stroke	disability	patent	reflex	obesity
blockage	anterior	associate	accident	circulation

1. Figure out a way where you could quickly have an apple _____ prove that this is a comfortable product.

2. Obesity correlates with increased risk for hypertension and _____.

3. The logical treatment is to remove this _____.

4. Even so, Japan's _____ has caused some political leaders to pause the progression of nuclear power.

5. When Julie speaks of her _____, she talks in the same calm, level tones she uses to discuss her A level prospects.

6. At this moment, there is no ocular _____.

7. The stroke caused by an _____ circulation large artery clots may be treated through operation.

8. This is _____ nonsense.

9. A number of forged banknote are in _____.

10. The World Health Organization calls _____ a global epidemic.

III. Supplementary

Text B

Parkinson Disease

Parkinson's disease (PD) is a type of movement disorder. It happens when nerve cells in the brain don't produce enough of dopamine. PD usually begins around age 60, but it can start earlier. It is more common in men than in women.

Pre-reading

1. What is Parkinson's disease?

2. What are the symptoms of Parkinson's disease?

3. What is DBS?

Parkinson's disease (PD) was first described by an English physician, James Parkinson in 1817 in "An Essay on the Shaking Palsy." the famous French neurologist, Charcot, further described the syndrome in the late 1800s. It is a type of movement disorder which happens when nerve cells in the brain don't produce enough of a brain chemical called dopamine.

ER-7-25
扫一扫 听一
听

A number of risk factors have been associated with an increased risk of PD, with age being the most important one. In addition to age, male gender and race, as well as positive family history may increase the risk for PD. A variety of environment exposure including herbicide and pesticide exposure, metals, drinking well water, farming, rural residence, wood pulp mills and steel alloy industries have been shown to increase the risk of PD. Finally, the life experiences (trauma, emotional stress, personality traits like shyness and depressiveness) may affect the risk, although this is less well proven. On the other hand, an inverse correlation between cigarette smoking and caffeine intake has been found in case-control studies, the significance of these correlations being however, unclear. Symptoms begin gradually, often on one side of the body. Later they affect both sides. They include:

ER-7-26
扫一扫 知情
节

Trembling of hands, arms, legs, jaw and face

Stiffness of the arms, legs and trunk

Slowness of movement

Poor balance and coordination

As symptoms get worse, people with the disease may have trouble walking, talking, or doing simple tasks. They may also have problems such as depression, sleep problems, or trouble chewing, swallowing, or speaking.

There is no lab test for PD, so it can be difficult to diagnose. Doctors use a medical history and a neurological examination to diagnose it.

There is no cure for PD. A variety of medicines sometimes help symptoms dramatically. Surgery and deep brain stimulation (DBS) can help severe cases. With DBS, electrodes are surgically implanted in the brain. They send electrical pulses to stimulate the parts of the brain that control movement. There's no standard treatment for the disease-the treatment for each person with Parkinson's is based on his or her symptoms. Treatments include medication and surgical therapy. Other treatments include lifestyle modifications like getting more rest and more exercise.

Nursing interventions include:

Assess neurological status.

Assess ability to swallow and chew.

Provide a high-calorie, high-protein, high-fiber soft diet with small, frequent feedings.

Increase fluid intake to 2000 ml/d.

Promote independence along with safety measures.

Avoid rushing the client with activities.

Promote physical therapy and rehabilitation.

Provide a firm mattress, and position the client prone, without a pillow, to facilitate proper posture.

Encourage the client to lift his or her feet when walk, etc.

(445words)

Words in Focus

palsy /ˈpɔlzi/	*n.*	麻痹，中风
neurologist /nuˈrɑːlədʒist/	*n.*	＜医＞神经病学家

笔记

dopamine /'doʊpəmiːn/	n.	＜生化＞多巴胺
gender /'dʒɛndə/	n.	性别
herbicide /'hɜːbisaid/	n.	除草剂
pesticide /'pɛsti‚said/	n.	杀虫剂，农药
inverse /in'vɜːs/	adj.	相反的，逆向的，倒转的
electrode /i'lektroʊd/	n.	电极，电焊条
implant /im'plænt/	vt.	植入，插入

Useful Expressions

| personality traits | 人格特质 |
| case-control study | 病例对照研究 |

Post-reading

I. Comprehension of the text

Ⅰ) **Choose the best answer to complete each sentence with the information from the text.**

1. "An Essay on the Shaking Palsy." is written by _____.

   A. James Parkinson   B. Charcot   C. an unknown doctor

2. Parkinson's disease (PD) happens when nerve cells in the brain don't produce enough of _____.

   A. hormone   B. insulin   C. dopamine

3. A number of risk factors, such as positive family history, environment exposure and _____ have been associated with an increased risk of PD.

   A. tobacco smoking

   B. age, male gender and race

   C. high blood cholesterol

4. Symptoms of PD begin gradually, often on _____. Later they affect both sides.

   A.one side of the leg   B.one side of the body   C. one side of the arm

5. "There is no cure for PD" means _____.

   A. A person may fully recover from PD after the treatment.

   B. A person may partially recover from PD after the treatment.

   C. A person can not be treated for suffering from PD.

Ⅱ) **Read the following statements and then decide whether each of them is true or false based on the information from the text. Write T for true and F for false in the space provided.**

_____ 1. Parkinson's disease is a type of movement disorder which happens when nerve cells in the brain don't produce enough of a brain chemical.

_____ 2. Age is the most important risk factor associated with PD.

_____ 3. Cigarette smoking and caffeine intake have an positive correlation to Parkinson's disease.

_____ 4. The treatment for each person with Parkinson's is based on his or her reasons.

II. Vocabulary activities

Find a word or phrase from the box below to complete each sentence. Change word forms where necessary.

| describe | addition | posture | affect | intake |
| exposure | inverse | modification | implant | prove |

1. Nowadays, I rarely ever work on my laptop as it encourages such a bad _____.
2. when the direct approach failed he tried the _____ one.
3. Your _____ is ready to deliver.
4. It is a matter of fact that excessive _____ to the sun's rays can cause skin cancer.
5. He worries about the other markets, but he refrains from using the word 'bubble' to _____ them.
6. A good teacher should _____ high ideals in children.
7. It's been very nice to _____ them wrong.
8. The air _____ must be silenced to some degree.
9. You never allow personal problems to _____ your performance.
10. In _____ to California, Nevada and Florida have passed laws allowing driverless cars to be tested within their borders.

III. Supplementary

ER-7-29
扫一扫 答案
"晓"

ER-7-30
扫一扫 练一
练

Part IV Writing

Writing a Nursing Assessment

Instructions:

Nursing Assessment is the first stage of the nursing process in which the nurse carries out a complete and holistic nursing assessment of every patient's needs. The purpose of this stage is to identify the patient's nursing problems. These problems are expressed as either actual or potential. For example, a patient who has been rendered immobile by a road traffic accident may be assessed as having the "potential for impaired skin integrity related to immobility".

A nursing assessment should includes a nursing history, psychological and social examination and physical examination. Taking a nursing history allows a nurse to establish a report with the patient and family. Elements of the history include: the client's overall health status, the course of the present illness including symptoms, the current management of illness, the client's medical history (including familial medical history), social history and how the client perceives his illness. The main areas considered in a psychological examination are intellectual health and emotional health. Assessment of cognitive function and checking for hallucinations and delusions, measuring concentration levels, and inquiring into the client's hobbies and interests constitute an intellectual health assessment. Emotional health is assessed by observing and inquiring about how the client feels and what he does in response to these feelings. Religion and beliefs are also important areas to consider. A physical examination includes the observation or measurement of signs, which can be observed or measured, or symptoms such as nausea or vertigo, which can be felt by the patient.

The assessment is documented in the patient's medical or nursing records, which may be on paper or as part of the electronic medical record.

A range of instruments has been developed to assist nurses in their assessment role. These include: the index of independence in activities of daily living, the Barthel index, the Creighton Royal behavior rating scale, the Clifton assessment procedures for the elderly, the general health

笔记

questionnaire, and the geriatric mental health state schedule. Other assessment tools may focus on a specific aspect of the patient's care.

For example, the water low score and the Braden scale deals with a patient's risk of developing a pressure ulcer , the Glasgow Coma Scale measures the conscious state of a person, and various pain scales.

Sentence Patterns:

中文护理证明常表达为有潜在的……风险，英语多译为"having the potential risk for... related to immobility."

A nursing assessment usually consists of the following parts:

1. **the heading** (nursing assessment)
2. **the body** (the main content of the nursing assessment)
3. **the signature** (hand written or typed)

Examples:

1. *Notes*

   a girl, 5 years old,

   Signs and symptoms: fever, nasal obstruction and a sore throat, persistent cough, Koplik's
   spots are present in the mouth, the lungs clear, moderate splenomegaly.

   History: in good health until about four days prior to admission, fever for the past few days,
   and today it was 103'F, no history of any recent measles contact

A five-year-old female was in good health until four days prior to admission. Then she began to sneeze and to complain of some nasal obstruction and a sore throat. Her cough was persistent. She has had a fever for the past 2 days, and today it was 103'F. There is no history of any recent measles contact.

On physical examination the vital signs were within normal limits, except for the temperature. Koplik's spots are present in the mouth. The lungs are clear, and there is moderate splenomegaly.

2. *Notes*

   A baby girl, 12 months old

   Symptoms: Sudden pain in abdomen, accompanied by nausea and vomiting

   History: Healthy until last night when the baby felt a sudden and acute pain in her abdomen,
   fever and cough developed this morning,

   Vomiting three times since this morning

   No stool this morning

The patient is a baby girl, one year old. She was hospitalized on Jan. 1, 2013. On admission her parents told that the baby had been healthy until last night when she suddenly felt a severe pain in her belly. She also felt nausea and vomited 3 times this morning. The baby developed a fever and a cough this morning. She had no stool this morning.

Practice:

Patient name:	*Alice Wang*
Sex:	*Female*
Occupation:	*clerk*
DOB:	*Jan, 14ᵗʰ, 1960*

笔记

Chief complaint: *Fever for two days, got worse today; Vomiting at home this morning*
History: *Mild headache Activity and appetite normal in the first few days Hand, foot and buttock rash noted for 4 days*

ER-7-31
扫一扫 答案
"晓"

Part V   Enriching your word power

1.	cephal(o)	头
	cephalodynia /ˈsefələdiniə/ 同 cephalalgia	头痛
	cephalotomy /ˌsefəˈlɔtəm/	胎头切开术，穿颅术
2.	cerebr(o)	大脑
	cerebroma /seriˈbrəumə/	脑瘤
	cerebrum /səˈriːbrəm/	大脑
3.	encephal(o)	脑
	hydrocephalic /haidrəuseˈfælik/	脑积水的
	encephalomyelitis /enˌsefələumaiəˈlaitis/	脑脊髓炎
4.	cerbell(o)	小脑
	cerebellum /ˌserəˈbeləm/	小脑
	cerebellospinal /seiəˈbelɒspinl/	小脑脊髓的
5.	crani(o)	颅骨，颅
	craniopuncture /kreiˈniːəupʌŋktʃər/	颅穿刺术
	craniology /ˌkreiniˈɒlədʒi/	颅骨学
6.	thalam(o)	丘脑
	thalamencephalon /ˌθæləmenˈsefəlɒn/	间脑，丘脑
	thalamic /θəˈlæmik/	丘脑的，视丘的
7.	neur(o)	神经
	neuroanatomy /ˌnjuərəuəˈnætəmi/	神经解剖学
	neuroglia /njuəˈrɒgliə/	神经胶质
8.	gangli(o)	神经节
	gangliocytoma /gangliocytoma/ 同 ganglioneuroma	神经节细胞瘤
	ganglioma /gæŋgliˈəumə/	神经节瘤
9.	gli(o)	胶质
	gliogenous /gˈlaiəudʒenəs/	胶质原的
	gliocytoma /glaiəsaiˈtəmə/ 同 glioma	胶质细胞瘤

笔记

107

10. mening(o); meningi(o)　　　　　　　　　　脑膜，脊膜
    meningitis /ˌmenin'dʒaitis/　　　　　　　脑膜炎
    meningoencephalitis /mi'niŋɡəʊənsefə'laitis/　脑膜脑炎

11. myel(o)　　　　　　　　　　　　　　　脊髓，骨髓
    myelitis /ˌmaiə'laitis/　　　　　　　　　脊髓炎
    myeloneuritis /maiələʊnjʊə'raitis/　　　脊髓神经炎

12. spin(o)　　　　　　　　　　　　　　　脊，棘，刺
    spinogram /spi'nəɡræm/　　　　　　　脊柱 X 线照片；脊髓造影照片
    spinous /'spainəs/　　　　　　　　　　多刺的，刺状的

13. hemi-; semi-　　　　　　　　　　　　半，偏，单侧
    hemianopia /ˌhemiən'əʊpiə/　　　　　偏盲
    semisupination /semisʌpi'neiʃn/　　　　半仰卧位

14. -lepsy　　　　　　　　　　　　　　　发作
    narcolepsy /'nɑ:kəʊlepsi/　　　　　　　嗜眠发作
    epilepsy /'epilepsi/　　　　　　　　　　癫痫症

15. phob(o)　　　　　　　　　　　　　　恐怖
    phobia /'fəʊbiə/　　　　　　　　　　　恐怖病，恐怖症
    acrophobia /ˌækrə'fəʊbiə/　　　　　　恐高症

16. phren(o)- ; psych(o)-; thym(o) -　　　精神，意志，情感
    phrenitic /fri'nitik/　　　　　　　　　　精神错乱的，精神病的
    psychotherapy /ˌsaikəʊ'θerəpi/　　　　精神疗法，心理疗法
    dysthymia /dis'θaimiə/　　　　　　　　心境恶劣，心情恶劣

17. schiz(o)-　　　　　　　　　　　　　分裂
    schizoaffective /skizəʊ'fektiv/　　　　　情感性分裂的
    schizophrenia /ˌskitsə'fri:niə/　　　　　精神分裂症

18. -mania　　　　　　　　　　　　　　异常冲动
    necromania /nekrəʊ'meiniə/　　　　　恋尸狂，恋尸癖

19. -asthenia　　　　　　　　　　　　　虚弱，无力
    neurasthenia /ˌnjʊərəs'θi:niə/　　　　　神经衰弱症

Part Ⅵ Exercise

Directions: *In this section, only one of the following options is correct, please choose.*

（刘清泉　吕小君）

ER-7-32
扫一扫 看一
看

笔 记

Unit 8
Urogenital Department

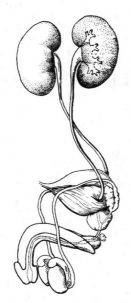

Fig. 8-1   urogenital department

Health is the most precious gift that nature can prepare for us the most fair.

健康是自然所能给我们准备的最公平最珍贵的礼物。

——Montaigne（蒙田）

Learning Objectives

Skill focus

1. *Master the way of answering the consultation from the patients.*

2. *Know how to give treatment for urinary diseases.*

3. *Understand the process of writing case history.*

Language focus

1. *Basic medical words and expressions when meeting patients with urinary diseases.*

2. *Have ability of creating and guessing a new word using roots and prefix or suffix.*

Part I   Listening

This section is designed to test your ability to understand spoken English in nursing or medical contexts. You will hear a selection of recorded materials and you must answer the questions that accompany them. There are TWO parts in this section, Part A and Part B.

Part A

Words in Focus

intravenous /ˌɪntrəˈviːnəs/	*adj.*	静脉注射的；进入静脉的
pyelography /paɪəˈlɒɡrəfi/	*n.*	肾盂造影术
hydronephrosis /ˌhaɪdrənɪˈfrəʊsɪs/	*n.*	肾盂积水
iodine /ˈaɪədiːn/	*n.*	碘
anaphylactic /ˌænəfɪˈlæktɪk/	*adj.*	过敏性的
hyperthyrosis /haɪpəθaɪəˈrəʊsɪs/	*n.*	甲状腺功能亢进
cachexia /kəˈkeksɪə/	*n.*	恶质病
malformation /ˌmælfɔːrˈmeɪʃn/	*n.*	畸形
hypotension /ˌhaɪpəˈtenʃən/	*n.*	低血压
numbness /ˈnʌmnəs/	*n.*	麻木

Useful Expressions

B-scan	B 超
renal function	肾功能
intravenous pyelography	静脉肾盂造影技术
acute nephritis	急性肾炎
acute pyelitis	急性肾盂炎
urinary stone	泌尿系结石
side effect	副作用
lower limbs	下肢

Text

Directions: *In this section you will hear a short passage, at the end of the passage, one or more questions will be asked about what was said, decide which the best answer is.*

Background:

A 53-year-old woman Mrs. Liu states 2 years history of increasing waist pain. Her B-scan shows that there is hydronephrosis on her left side kidney. In order to examine the renal function, she may need to receive intravenous pyelography examination. She is inquiring Doctor Wang whether she is fit for receiving the intravenous pyelography examination.

Comprehension of the Text

1. Mrs. Liu has already finished her B-scan.

   A. Yes.   B. No.   C. Not mentioned.

2. According to the dialogue, what kind of problem does Mrs. Liu have now?

   A. She has severe heart disease.

   B. She has urinary stone.

   C. She has hydronephrosis on the left side kidney.

3. According to the dialogue, which of the following statements is true?

   A. Patient with acute nephritis should receive intravenous pyelography.

   B. Patient with urinary stone should receive renal intravenous pyelography.

   C. Patient with heart disease should receive renal intravenous pyelography.

4. Is there any side effects according to Doctor Wang?

A. Yes.   B. No.   C. Not mentioned.

5. According to the dialogue, what side effect does the intravenous pyelography have?

    A. heart attack   B. hydronephrosis   C. abdominal pain

Part B

Words in Focus

urinary /'jʊərinri/	*adj.*	泌尿的；尿的
persistent /pər'sistənt/	*adj.*	持久稳固的
micturition /ˌmiktjʊ'riʃn/	*n.*	排尿
sample /'sæmpl/	*n.*	样品；样本
bacteriuria /bækˌtiəri'jʊəriə/	*n.*	菌尿
amoxicillin /əmɒksə'silin/	*n.*	羟氨苄青霉素；阿莫西林

ER-8-5
扫一扫 读一读

Useful Expressions

urinary tract infection	尿路感染；尿道发炎
pass urine	小便
frequent micturition	尿频
urgent micturition	尿急
burning pain	灼痛；烧痛
burning sensation	烧灼感
urine test	尿检
clear out	清除；（使）离开

ER-8-6
扫一扫 看一看

Text

Directions: *In this section you will hear a short passage, at the end of the passage, one or more questions will be asked about what was said, decide which the best answer is.*

Background:

    The following conversation is about urinary tract infection. Mrs. White is stating her symptoms to Doctor Smith on Wednesday in doctor's office. She has some problems when she passes urine and she wants to find some treatments from Doctor Smith. Please listen to the conversation carefully and choose the right answer for each question.

ER-8-7
扫一扫 听一听

Comprehension of the text

1. Mrs. White has some problems when she passes urine.

    A. Yes.   B. No.   C. Not mentioned.

2. How many times does Mrs. White have to get up at night?

    A. four or five times   B. three or five times   C. twice or three times

3. What kind of feeling does Mrs. White have when she urinates?

    A. She feels like it is the same as it used to be.

    B. She feels like burning sensation and not as good as it used to be.

    C. She feels like there is still a good strong flow.

4. How does Doctor Smith make the definite diagnosis?

    A. by asking the symptoms of the patient

    B. by referring the result of the urine test

    C. by inquiring the symptoms of the patient and read the urine test as reference

ER-8-8
扫一扫 知情节

笔记

111

5. What's the treatment from Doctor Smith?

    A. Asking the patient to drink more water.

    B. Prescribing antibiotics such as amoxicillin to clear out the infection.

    C. Asking the patient to drink plenty of coffee, and soft drinks.

Part Ⅱ   Speaking

This section is designed to test your speaking ability. After learning the following conversation A and B you will have the ability of speaking skill in medical and nursing working and try to do the following speaking tasks.

Conversation 1

Acute Pyelonephritis

ER-8-9
扫一扫 听一听

ER-8-10
扫一扫 知情节

Doctor Vincent is inquiring the patient Mrs. Robert's condition in the office. Mrs. Robert is about 50 years old and has a good physical condition in daily life. Nevertheless recently she feels uncomfortable, especially when she urinates. Doctor Vincent asks her some questions and then makes a definite diagnosis.

Dr. Vincent:	Good morning, Mrs. Robert. What brings you here today?
Mrs. Robert:	Well, I have been feeling pain when urinating.
Dr. Vincent:	How long have you had it?
Mrs. Robert:	It started two weeks ago.
Dr. Vincent:	OK. What kind of pain is it?
Mrs. Robert:	Oh...I think it's a kind of burning sensation. And now it seems to be getting worse, I have to pee every half hour or so, and I have to rush to go to the toilet.
Dr. Vincent:	OK...as you mentioned, there are frequent micturition and urgent micturition... any other symptoms?
Mrs. Robert:	Well... Also, I think I have a terrible headache and lumbago. Sometimes I feel feverish or shivery. And it seems that I have trouble getting started.
Dr. Vincent:	Oh, that's the symptoms of high fever, chills, and dysuria I think. How many times do you have to pass urine at night?
Mrs. Robert:	I can't say, anyway, several times every night.
Dr. Vincent:	Do you have any blood in your urine?
Mrs. Robert:	No. I don't.
Dr. Vincent:	Is your urine turbid?
Mrs. Robert:	Oh, yes, I think I have urine turbidity.
Dr. Vincent:	Well, based on your description, I suppose you may have an acute pyelonephritis, a kind of urinary tract infection. But I think we still need a routine urinalysis before making a definite diagnosis.
Mrs. Robert:	OK. I understand.
Dr. Vincent:	Now would you please go to the washroom and provide some urine sample in this cup?

笔记

Mrs. Robert: Sure.

(One hour later, Mrs. Robert meets Doctor Vincent again in his office.

Dr. Vincent: Mrs. Robert, according to the routine urinalysis, the bacteria have entered your bladder and your kidneys. Therefore, we need to treat it promptly in case it becomes worse.

Mrs. Robert: Hum, I know. So what kind of treatment you'll give me?

Dr. Vincent: You need an injection and also some tablets like antibiotics. At the same time, you should rest in bed and drink plenty of water.

Mrs. Robert: OK, Do I need to come back and see you again?

Dr. Vincent: Yes. I'd like to see you in five days. If you feel worse, come to the emergency clinic immediately.

Mrs. Robert: Great! Thank you so much for all of the information. You have been very helpful.

Dr. Vincent: Never mind it. I hope you'll recover quickly.

Mrs. Robert: Thank you, see you next time.

Dr. Vincent: See you.

(375 words)

Words in Focus

pyelonephritis /paɪələʊniˈfraɪtɪs/	*n.*	肾盂肾炎
scalding /ˈskɔldɪŋ/	*adj.*	滚烫的，灼热的
pee /piː/	*vi.*	小便；撒尿
lumbago /lʌmˈbeɪgəʊ/	*n.*	腰痛
chills /tʃɪls/	*n.*	寒冷（chill 的名词复数）
dysuria /disˈjʊərɪə/	*n.*	排尿困难
turbid /ˈtɜːbid/	*adj.*	混浊的
kidney /ˈkidni/	*n.*	肾；肾脏
tablet /ˈtæblit/	*n.*	药片

Useful Expressions

physical condition	身体状况；健康水平
urine turbidity	尿浊度
routine urinalysis	尿常规
emergency clinic	急诊

ER-8-11
扫一扫 读一读

ER-8-12
扫一扫 看一看

I. Free talk

Directions: *Work in pairs and discuss the following questions after learning to the recording of Dialogue One.*

1. Based on the conversation, describe to your desk mate the symptoms of acute pyelonephritis.

_____

_____

2. According to the conversation, discuss with your desk mate what should a patient do if she got an acute pyelonephritis, what kind of treatment should the doctor give to the patient ?

_____

_____

笔记

II. Make a dialogue

Directions: *Work in pairs, play the parts of Chinese nurse and Chinese patient separately, and try to make a short dialogue related to acute pyelonephritis.*

ER-8-13
扫一扫 答案
"晓"

> **Sample Dialogue:**
>
> Nurse Li: Good afternoon. I am nurse Li. Can I help you?
>
> Patient Sun: Good afternoon. Nurse Li. I feel tired and aching and I also feel uncomfortable when I urinate recently.
>
> Nurse Li: It seems that there's a problem with your urinary system.
>
> Patient Sun: ...

Conversation 2

Nephritis

ER-8-14
扫一扫 听一
听

Sam is an intern, he works in urology department. Mrs. Kate is a 50-year-old patient. She doesn't feel very well recently, and she feels pain in her waist for a long time, even if she has edema on her eyelids. Therefore, she comes to the hospital and consults intern Sam. After doing investigation and inspection, Sam gives diagnosis and suggestions to Kate.

ER-8-15
扫一扫 知情
节

Intern Sam:	Good morning, Mrs. Kate. What seems to be the problem?
Mrs. Kate:	Well, I always feel tired, weakness, and pain in my waist recently, and I also find that I have edema on my eyelids, face and ankle... especially in the morning these days...I don't know what's wrong with me.
Intern Sam:	OK, When did it start?
Mrs. Kate:	Well...I think maybe it started one week ago.
Intern Sam:	How about your urination? Is it the same as before?
Mrs. Kate:	No, the urine is small in quantity actually, and the color seems to be dark and it has a lot of foam.
Intern Sam:	How many times do you have to pass urine at night?
Mrs. Kate:	I have to pee 3 to 4 times, while I didn't do that before.
Intern Sam:	Do you have hematuria?
Mrs. Kate:	Yes, I do.
Intern Sam:	How about the shortness of breath lately?
Mrs. Kate:	Err...no. I don't have it. Actually I caught cold two weeks ago and I have had a sore throat till now, but no shortness of breath.
Intern Sam:	Have you take some medicine?
Mrs. Kate:	No, I haven't.
Intern Sam:	OK, how old are you?
Mrs. Kate:	50.
Intern Sam:	Now let me take your blood pressure. Oh, 150/100mmHg, hypertension, of course. Would you please open your mouth and stick your tongue out? I want to examine your throat, oh...enlargement of the amygdala (3rd degrees).
Mrs. Kate:	OK, that's why I feel sore throat.

笔 记

Intern Sam:　Yes, please show me your limbs and let me check them. Alright, you see, you get edema of the lower limbs.

Mrs. Kate:　So, doctor, what is wrong with me ?

Intern Sam:　I can't give the definite diagnosis until we do some physical examination. Please take a routine urinalysis, and then we'll talk about the diagnosis and treatment.

(30 minutes later)

Mrs. Kate:　Here is the urine test report.

Intern Sam:　OK, you have proteinuria and hematuria, and the index of urine samples is abnormal. I think it's appropriate to diagnose your disease to be 'acute nephritis' at present.

Mrs. Kate:　Acute nephritis? Is it serious?

Intern Sam:　I've just finished talking to other doctor. We both think you should go through the admission procedures immediately.

Mrs. Kate:　Oh... all right. Thank you, doctors.

Intern Sam:　Don't mention it. Would you just wait here for a few minutes? I'll get a nurse to take care of you.

Mrs. Kate:　OK, thank you.

ER-8-16
扫一扫 读一读

(369 words)

ER-8-17
扫一扫 看一看

Words in Focus

edema /iˈdiːmə/	n.	浮肿；水肿
eyelids /ˈailids/	n.	眼睑
urination /ˌjuəriˈneiʃən/	n.	排尿
amygdala /əˈmigdələ/	n.	扁桃体结构
hematuria /ˌhiːməˈtjuəriə/	n.	尿血；血尿症
proteinuria /ˌprəutiːˈnuərˈiːə/	n.	蛋白尿
index /ˈinˌdɛks/	n.	指数
admission /ædˈmiʃən/	n.	承认；准许进入

Useful Expressions

physical examination　　　　　　　　　　　体检

I. Free talk

Directions: Work in pairs and discuss the following questions after learning to the Dialogue Two

1. What is the physical condition with patient Kate?

_____

_____

2. What has been done by intern Sam in order to make a definite diagnosis for patient Kate's disease?

_____

_____

3. What's the result of Kate's urinalysis?

_____

_____

笔记

4. Suppose you are intern Sam, after giving reception to patient Kate, you try to make a conclusion about receiving patient with nephritis, from the aspects of receiving patient, diagnosing, giving treatment, prevention, and pacifying patient.

_____

_____

II. Comprehension of the text

Directions: According to the conversation and complete the sentences

1. Fatigue, weakness, _____, _____, and pain in the waist are all symptoms of Nephritis.

   A. edema on eyelids, hematuria

   B. coughing, sneezing

   C. proteinuria, cough

2. The routine urinalysis can give us data about _____ and _____.

   A. enlargement of the amygdala, blood pressure

   B. proteinuria, hematuria

   C. enlargement of the amygdala, and hematuria

3. _____ can prove that the urine sample is abnormal.

   A. hematuria

   B. edema of the lower limbs

   C. enlargement of amygdala

4. According to Sam, _____ is hypertension.

   A. 150/100mmHg   B. 120/80mmHg   C. 135/85mmHg

5. If the patient was diagnosed as acute nephritis, the best way for patient to receive treatment is _____.

   A. going back home and having a sleep

   B. applying for hospital admission and being hospitalized for observation

   C. taking drugs and drinking more water, but don't need to have a rest

Part III   Reading

Text A

> As a part of body's circulatory system, kidneys filter the blood, get rid of waste products, control the blood pressure, and stimulate the production of red blood cells. However, if kidneys lost their function, it is called kidney failure. What do you know about kidney failure? We will learn it in this part.
>
> ### Pre-reading
> 1. What is the location of kidneys?
> 2. How many kinds of kidney failure in medicine?

Kidney Failure

There are two kidneys in human body. They are two bean-shaped organs. They are located at the back of the upper abdomen of the human body, on either side of the spine. As a part of body's circulatory system, kidneys expel toxin, filter the blood and produce the urine. Once the kidneys lost their function, some terrible kidney disease would appear. The end-stage of kidney disease or kidney's losing function is called kidney failure.

Kidney failure can be divided into acute kidney failure and chronic kidney failure. Acute kidney failure is a sudden loss of kidney's ability to perform their main function. Chronic kidney failure is a gradual loss of kidney function over time.

Acute kidney failure is reversible on the condition that the patient's physical condition is healthy. But if the patient he himself got some chronic disease, like high blood pressure, diabetes, kidney stones, and prostate disease, and be given inadequately treatments, permanent damage or chronic renal failure may occur. Signs and symptoms of acute kidney failure may include: decreased urine output, shortness of breath, fatigue, metabolic disorder, edema, etc.

Chronic kidney failure is a progressive, irreversible deterioration of kidney function. In clinic, it is asymptomatic in the early stage of chronic kidney failure. As the disease becomes worse, the diseased kidney will lose its function of expelling toxin. In the final stage: with the toxic substances in the blood increasing continuously, uremia would appear.

Acute kidney failure is most common in people who are already hospitalized, particularly people who need intensive care. As for chronic kidney failure, it is most common in patient who has acute renal failure, who has metabolic disease or damage of renal blood vessels due to hypertension or diabetes, etc.

Diagnosis of kidney failure is confirmed by blood tests measuring the buildup of waste products in the blood. Nursing goals and interventions for acute kidney failure are similar to that of chronic kidney failure. We can treat kidney failure by methods of controlling diet, using medication, giving dialysis, and kidney transplantation.

On nursing, for patient with kidney failure, diet is an important consideration. They should consult dietitian and get some suggestions about what kind of food may or may not be appropriate. Medication may be used for helping control some issues associated with kidney failure. As for dialysis, there are hemodialysis and peritoneal dialysis. In one word, once kidney failure appeared, people should prevent further deterioration of renal losing function, just in case the appearance of complete kidney failure.

(412 words)

Words in Focus

spine /spaɪn/	n.	脊柱；脊椎
filter /'fɪltə/	vt.	过滤
diabetes /ˌdaɪə'biːtis, -tiz/	n.	糖尿病；多尿症
prostate /'prɑːsteit/	n.	前列腺
reversible /ri'vɜːsibl/	adj.	可逆的；可医治的
deterioration /diˌtɪəriə'reiʃn/	n.	恶化；退化
toxic /'tɒksik/	adj.	有毒的；中毒的
uremia /juə'riːmiə/	n.	尿毒症
hospitalize /'hɒspitəlaiz/	vt.	把……送入医院治疗
dialysis /ˌdai'æləsis/	n.	透析

ER-8-21
扫一扫 读一读

ER-8-22
扫一扫 看一看

笔记

Useful Expressions

expel toxin   排毒

metabolic disorder   代谢障碍，代谢紊乱

intensive care   重病特别护理

acute kidney failure   急性肾衰竭

chronic kidney failure   慢性肾衰竭

hemodialysis   血液透析

peritoneal dialysis   腹膜透析

Post-reading

I. Comprehension of the text

Ⅰ) Choose the best answer to complete each sentence with the information from the text.

1. Usually there are _____ kidneys in our body, and they are _____ shaped organs.

   A. two, bean   B. one, round   C. three, box

2. Kidney failure can be divided into _____ Kidney failure or _____ Kidney Failure.

   A. a benign, malignant   B. a fast, slow   C. an acute, chronic

3. Chronic kidney failure is a progressive, irreversible deterioration of kidney function.

   A. Yes   B. No   C. Not mentioned

4. Diagnosis of kidney failure is based on _____.

   A. electrolyte   B. blood tests   C. diabetes

5. For people with kidney failure, they don't need to consider their diet and also they don't need to consult a dietitian.

   A. yes   B. no   C. not mentioned

Ⅱ) Read the following statements and then decide whether each of them is true or false based on the information from the text. Write T for true and F for false in the space provided.

_____ 1. Acute kidney failure refers to the gradual loss of kidney function.

_____ 2. Acute kidney failure is most common in people who are already hospitalized, particularly people who need intensive care.

_____ 3. High blood pressure, diabetes can cause kidney failure.

_____ 4. For patient with kidney failure, diet is not an important consideration.

II. Vocabulary activities

Find a word or phrase from the box below to complete each sentence. Change word forms where necessary.

filter	circulatory	dialysis	interventions	metabolic
diabetes	toxic	reversible	asymptomatic	abdomen

1. Nursing goals and _____ for acute kidney failure are similar to that of chronic kidney failure.

2. Kidney is one organ in our body; it is belonged to _____ system.

3. Symptoms of acute kidney failure may include: decreased urine output, shortness of breath, fatigue, _____ disorder.

4. The function of kidney is to _____ the blood and to get rid of the metabolic wastes.

5. _____, high blood pressure, and kidney stones are the common causes for kidney failure.

6. Besides medication, _____ is a conventional therapy for those with kidney failure.

7. Kidneys are the same size as man's fist, and it's located at the back of people's upper _____ .

8. Acute kidney failure is _____ on the condition that the patient's physical condition is healthy.

9. The _____ substances in the blood increasing continuously, uremia would appear.

10. In clinic, it is _____ in the early stage of chronic kidney failure.

III. Supplementary

Text B

> Kidney transplantation is a surgical operation. When patient' kidneys lost their function of expelling toxin completely, which is also called kidney failure, kidney transplantation would be the best treatment for the patient.
>
> ### Pre-reading
> 1. What is the definition of kidney transplantation?
> 2. What are do's and don'ts after kidney transplantation?

Kidney Transplantation

Kidney transplantation is a surgical operation, in which the doctor will transplant a kidney, from a live or cadaver donor, into a recipient whose kidneys can no longer function properly. When kidneys losing their ability of eliminating excess fluid build-up and metabolic wastes from blood—which is known as kidney failure or the end-stage kidney disease—kidney transplantation would be suggested to be the best treatment. Compared with kidney from cadaver donor, kidney from well-matched living donor provides more chance for successful transplantation.

In kidney transplantation. The surgeon will not remove the diseased kidney from the patient. He will make a cut, which is about 15cm, on the left or right lower abdomen of the patient. He will place the new kidney inside the patient's lower abdomen; and ensure that the arteries and veins of the new kidney fit together with the large arteries and veins of the recipient. Once the doctor makes sure that there is blood flow to the kidney, the transplanted kidney will be placed in the iliac fossa, and the wound will be closed. Postoperative nursing management is necessary for hemostasis until the newly transplanted kidney functions well in the recipient's body.

After kidney transplantation, the patient may have complications, such as failure of the transplantation, rejection of the transplantation, infection, heart attack, stroke, as well as anti-rejection medication side effects. Therefore, the patient needs to take some medicine to prevent his or her body from rejecting the donor kidney.

Six hours after the operation, the patient should keep lying on bed without pillow, and this will last for 4 ～7 days. In order to avoid the renal rupture, the patient should also keep the lateral position, can not sit up, and can not bend lower limb of the transplanted kidney side. After one week or so, the patient can sit back, get out of the bed, and weight himself, but the action should be gentle. If the patient feels pain while doing exercise, he should stop activity immediately and report to the doctor.

1～2 days after the operation, the patient can eat some liquid food such as rice, egg soup. On the following day, the patient can eat semi-liquid food, and then normal food. The food should be low salt, low sugar, low fat, high vitamin and protein (animal protein). Also the diet should be easy to be digested, clean and fresh. Nourishing food such as ginseng and royal jelly should not be provided to the patient.

(448 words)

Words in Focus

surgical /'sɜːrdʒikl/	*adj.*	外科的；外科手术的
cadaver /kə'dævə/	*n.*	尸体
donor /'dounə(r)/	*n.*	捐赠者；供血者
recipient /ri'sɪpiənt/	*n.*	接受者
eliminate /ɪ'limi,neit/	*vt.*	淘汰；排除
Iliac fossa /'ili,æk 'fɑsə/	*n.*	髂窝
postoperative /,pəust'ɒpərətiv/	*adj.*	手术后的
hemostasis /hi'mɒstəsis/	n.	止血；止血法
rupture /'rʌptʃə/	n.	断裂；破裂
decubitus /di'kjuːbitəs/	n.	卧位；卧姿
vitamin /'vaitəmin/	n.	维生素
protein /'prouti:n/	n.	蛋白质
nourishing /'nʌriʃiŋ/	*adj.*	有营养的；滋养多的
ginseng /'dʒin,sɛŋ/	n.	人参

Useful Expressions

royal jelly	蜂王浆

Post-reading

I. Comprehension of the text

Read the following statements and then decide whether each of them is true or false based on the information from the text. Write T for true and F for false in the space provided.

_____ 1. It is reasonable to conclude from Paragraph 1 that kidney transplantation would be the best treatment for the patient if the patient lost their kidney function completely.

_____ 2. In the kidney surgery, the surgeon will remove the patient's diseased kidney at first, and then put the new kidney inside the patient's abdomen.

_____ 3. After kidney transplantation, the patient may have complications such as renal rejection, infection, heart attack, stroke as well as diabetes.

_____ 4. Patient should keep lying on bed and can eat nothing until 3 days later.

II. Vocabulary activities

Find a word or phrase from the box below to complete each sentence. Change word forms where necessary.

surgical	eliminate	postoperative	cadaver	rupture
complications	vitamin	recipient	exhaust	nourishing

ER-8-27
扫一扫 读一读

ER-8-28
扫一扫 看一看

笔记

1. The food given to the patient who were performed the kidney transplantation should be full of _____ and protein.

2. _____ food like ginseng, royal jelly, should not be supplied to the patient.

3. Kidney transplantation is a _____ operation.

4. She was too _____ and distressed to talk about the tragedy.

5. One of the kidney functions is to _____ the waste material from blood.

6. The _____ of kidney transplantation should express thanks and gratitude to the kidney donor.

7. After kidney transplantation, _____ nursing is necessary for maintaining hemostasis.

8. The patient should keep lying position and can not do aggravating activities in case there is kidney _____.

9. Usually kidney from a living donor is easier to be accepted by the patient, compared with the kidney from _____ donor.

10. About 1000 women die from childbirth-related _____ around the world every day.

III. Supplementary

ER-8-29
扫一扫 答案
"晓"

ER-8-30
扫一扫 练一
练

Part Ⅳ　Writing

Writing a Case History

Instructions:

　　The term case history and medical record are used to describe the systematic document of a single patient's medical history recorded by a doctor or other health care professionals. It includes both out-patient and in-patient records. Nowadays, we have Electronic Medical Record(EMR) and paper medical record. Here we mainly talked about paper medical record. It should contain sufficient information such as letters, symbols, charts and images etc so as to identify the patient, to support the diagnosis, and to justify the treatment.

　　We usually collect materials of case history by inquiring, physical check-ups, diagnoses, treatments, nursing, etc. The case history should be objective, based on real facts, accurate, timely completely, and standard. Usually, we write it by using a pen with black or blue ink. The languages used must be standard medical language; the expression should be accurate and the letters should be easily recognizable. In a word, the case history should be written according to some rules and signed by registered relative staff of the hospital.

　　When we write a case history, it should include several detailed items as below:

1. Personal details（个人基本情况）

2. Personal past medical history(PMH) include（个人史）

    Surgical history（外科手术史）

    Obstetric history (If the patient is a female, it is necessary)（婚育史）

    Drug history（用药史）

    Immunization history（免疫接种史）

3. Family history（家族史）

笔 记

121

4. Social history（社会史）

5. Chief complaint（主诉）

    Patient ideas, concerns and expectations

    （病人对疾病的陈述担心及渴望得到的治疗）

    History of the present illness（现病史）

6. Physical examination（体格检查）

7. Assessment and plan（初步诊断及治疗计划）

8. Give Orders and prescriptions（处方）

9. Signature of the relative doctors（主治医生签名）

Sentence Patterns:

When you write the chief complaint, sentence is composed of symptoms and time, without character name,article, and you should write it in the following patterns:

1. symptoms + for+ time（症状 +for+ 时间）:

    Chest pain for 2 hours 胸痛 2 小时

2. symptoms + of + time（症状 +of+ 时间）:

    Nausea and vomiting of three-day's duration 恶心呕吐 3 天

3. symptoms + time+in duration（症状 + 时间）:

    Headache 1 month in duration 头痛 1 个月

4. time + of +symptoms（时间 +of+ 症状）:

    Two-day history of fever 发热 2 天

Examples:

Case History

1. Personal details（个人基本情况）

    Surname: You sheng   First name: Chen

    Age: 50   Gender: male

    Marital Status: married   Occupation: Worker

    Race/nationality: Han/ China   Habit: Smoke frequently

    Date of Admission: 2011-12-31   Date of Record: 2011-12-31

2. Personal past medical history (PMH)（既往史）

    (Notes: It should include surgical history（外科手术史）, obstetric history（婚育史）, drug history（用药史）, immunization history（免疫接种史）

    Denied history of tuberculosis or viral hepatitis, diabetes mellitus, hypertension, endemic disease etc.

    Denied history of trauma, surgery, blood transfusion, intoxication etc.

    Denied food or drug Allergy. Denied history of long-term medication.

    Review of Systems(ROS).

3. Family history（家族史）:

    Both parents healthy and robust.

    Denied similar conditions among any family members.

    Denied history of infectious disease among family members.

笔 记

Denied familial history of complex disease.

4. Social history（个人史）：

Birth history: full term, uncomplicated vaginal delivery; no sign of neonatal distress.

Feeding history: good appetite and not picky at food.

Developmental history: mental and physical development equivalent to boys of the same age.

Life style: born and raised in the same place; he traveled to Japan on July 2011 before symptoms appeared. denied history of accessing infectious source; denied history of radiation, intoxication; Denied illicit drug use or alcohol consumption.

5. Chief complaint（主诉）：

(1) Patient ideas, concerns and expectations（病人对疾病的陈述、担心及渴望得到的治疗）：

Transient edema of both legs, edema of both eyelid for 2 month.

Worrying that he may get some fatal illness, and want to make sure what kind of disease he get.

(2) History of the present illness（现病史）：

February 2011, Chen developed edema of both legs with no cause. He denied fever, rash, hematuria, foamed urine and left it untreated. Symptoms relieved spontaneously 1 month later. May 2011, Chen complained of edema of both eyelids with no cause. He found it in the morning and the symptoms relieved in the afternoon without any complications. September 10 th 2011, he went to the local hospital for epigastric malaise and do physical check up. August 23 th 2011, Chen was transferred to our hospital. Chen is now admitted for further diagnosis and treatment.

6. Physical examination（体格检查）：

T 36.5℃　　　　HR 80 bpm　　　　RR 22/min　　　　Bp 123/70mmHg

Ht 179.0cm　　Wt 72.5kg　　BMI 23kg/m^2　　eGFR(EPI) 136.62ml/min

General survey: N(Normal)

Skin: N (Normal)

HEENT (Head, eye, ear, nose, throat): N (Normal)

Pulmonary: N (Normal)

Heart: N (Normal)

Peripheral vascular system: N(Normal)

Abdomen: N (Normal)

Urology system: Suspected kidney stone

Rectal and genitalia: N(Normal)

Extremities and musculoskeletal: N(Normal)

Neurologic: N(Normal)

7. Assessment and plan（初步诊断及治疗计划）：

I. Assessment

Based on the case history and all kinds of physical examination information,

Firstly, we should exclude the secondary and inherited glomerular diseases.

We may exclude infectious disease.

We may exclude autoimmune diseases for the moment.

We may exclude metabolic diseases by examining his ocular fundus.

We may exclude glomerular deposition diseases.

We may exclude drugs induced diseases.

Secondly, we consider the primary glomerular diseases. Renal biopsy is very important on this patient and the pathology may help make the decision of diagnosis and treatment.

Ⅱ. Plan

Do additional tests for diagnosis & differentials.

Give medication and support.

Contact the patient and prepare for a renal biopsy if possible.

Educate the patient and prepare for any possible complications and events.

Supervisor consultation.

8. Give orders and prescriptions（处方）:

1) Routine lab test including CBC, coagulation, urine and stool routine, liver & kidney function, infectious agents screening, ECG, 24h-UP, B-US for renal vessels and internal organs, monitoring BP, I/O and electrocytes, ocular fundus examination.

2) Predinisone 60mg po qd with Azathioprine 100mg Po qd, Calcitriol 0.25μg Po qd with Calcium carbonante tablets 500mg Po tid, Lipitor 10mg Po qn.

3) Prepare for a renal biopsy if possible.

9. Signature of the relative doctors（主治医生签名）:

Amy Yang

2011-12-3

(933 words)

Practice:

王女士，53 岁，已婚，教师，无不良生活习惯，作息规律。近一年的时间有身体不适的感觉，出现尿急、尿频、血尿、乏力、嗜睡、浮肿等症状，分别于 2013 年 3 月、5 月、9 月前往省立医院三次就诊并做检查，症状及病情出现反复，现到北京第一医科大学附属医院就诊，做了一系列检查，并试图查明病因。刘大夫现为王女士写了一份详细的病例记录。

_____

_____

_____

_____

_____

_____

_____

_____

_____

笔记

ER-8-31
扫一扫 答案
"晓"

Part Ⅴ   Enriching your word power

1. nephr(o)-; ren(o)- 肾
    nephritis /niˈfraitis/ 肾炎
    renopathy /ˈrinəpəθi/ 同 nephropathy 肾病

2. glomerul(o)- 肾小球
    glomerulonephritis /gləumerjuləunefˈraitis/ 肾小球性肾炎
    glomerulosclerosis /glɒmrjuləuskləˈrəusis/ 肾小球硬化症

3. pyel(o)- 肾盂
    pyelography /paiəˈlɒgrəfi/ 肾盂造影术
    pyelonephritis /paiələuniˈfraitis/ 肾盂肾炎

4. ureter(o)- 输尿管
    ureterolysis /juəriːtəˈrɒlisis/ 输尿管松解术
    ureterolithiasis /juə,riːtərɔliˈθaiəsis/ 输尿管石病

5. cyst(o)- 膀胱，囊，囊肿
    cystoadenoma /sistəudeˈnəumə/ 同 cystadenoma 囊腺瘤
    cystocele /ˈsistəsiːl/ 膀胱突出症

6. urethr(o)- 尿道
    urethrocystitis /juə,riːθrɔsisˈtaitis/ 尿道膀胱炎
    urethrostenosis /juəriːθrəstiˈnəusis/ 尿道狭窄

7. urin(o)-; ur(o)- 尿
    urinemia /juəriˈniːmiə/ 同 uremia 尿毒症
    uroclepsia /juərəuˈklepsjə/ 遗尿，尿失禁

8. lith(o)- 结石
    litholysis /laiˈtɒləsis/ 结石溶解
    lithureteria /liθjuriˈtiəriə/ 输尿管结石病

9. chyl(o)- 乳糜
    chylocyst /kaiˈləsist/ 同 cisterna chyli 乳糜池
    chyluria /ʃaiˈluəriə/ 乳糜尿，称 galacturia

10. gen(o)- 生殖，性
    genitoplasty /ˌdʒenitəuˈplɑːsti/ 生殖器成形术
    genohormone /dʒenəˈhɔːməun/ 基因激素

笔记

11.　andr(o)-　　　　　　　　　　　　　　　　　　男，雄
　　　androgen /'ændrədʒən/　　　　　　　　　　男性荷尔蒙，男性激素
　　　androgyne /ænd'rɒdʒain/　　　　　　　　　阴阳人，具有雌雄两性的花
12.　sperm(o)-; soermat(o)-　　　　　　　　　　　精液，精子
　　　spermatoblast /'spɜ:mətəublɑ:st/　　　　　精细胞，精子细胞
　　　spermocytoma /spɜ:mə'sitəmə/ 同 seminoma　精原细胞瘤

Part Ⅵ　Exercise

Directions: *In this section, only one of the following options is correct, please choose.*

（孙延宁　吕小君）

ER-8-32
扫一扫 看一看

笔 记

Unit 9
Obstetrics and Gynecology Department

Diet cures more than doctors.

自己饮食有节，胜过上门求医。

Part I   Listening

This section is designed to test your ability to understand spoken English in nursing or medical contexts. You will hear a selection of recorded materials and you must answer the questions that accompany them. There are TWO parts in this section, Part A and Part B.

ER-9-1
扫一扫 读一读

Part A

Words in Focus

pregnant /ˈpregnənt/	*adj.*	怀孕的
pregnancy /ˈpregnənsi/	*n.*	怀孕，妊娠
urine /ˈjuərin/	*n.*	尿，小便
prenatal /ˌpriːˈneitl/	*adj.*	出生前的，胎儿期的
menstrual /ˈmenstruəl/	*adj.*	月经的

ER-9-2
扫一扫 看一看

Useful Expressions

menstrual period	月经期
throw up	放弃，呕吐
a urine pregnancy test	一个尿妊娠试验
urine specimen	尿液样本
morning sickness	孕吐

笔记

ER-9-3
扫一扫 听一
听

ER-9-4
扫一扫 知情
节

Text

Directions: *In this section you will hear a short dialogue, please fill in the missing part according to what you here.*

Background:

Dr. Green is seeing patient Mrs. Baker, who wonders if she is pregnant.

Dr. Green:	Good morning, Mrs. Baker.
Mrs. Baker:	Good morning, Dr. Green.
Dr. Green:	1. _____
Mrs. Baker:	I missed my menstrual period. It was due 10 days ago, I wonder if I am pregnant.
Dr. Green:	When did you have your last period?
Mrs. Baker:	It was on November 21st.
Dr. Green:	How have you been feeling recently?
Mrs. Baker:	I think I'm having morning sickness because I feel like throwing up 2. _____. And I don't feel like eating anything, either, for a couple of days.
Dr. Green:	OK, well, I think you need to do a urine pregnancy test. Nurse Jackie will give you a specimen cup. Please come to see me with the result.
Mrs. Baker:	OK, thanks.
Nurse Jackie:	Mrs. Baker, here is the specimen cup with your name on it. 3. _____, the Ladies' Room is over there. Please come back to me with the cup filled halfway.
Mrs. Baker:	OK, thank you. (5 minutes later) Hi, Jackie, here is my urine specimen.
Nurse Jackie:	OK, I got it. Please take a seat in the waiting room.
Mrs. Baker:	All right! Thank you. How long will it take for the result to come out?
Nurse Jackie:	It should be here in 10 minutes. 4. _____ as soon as I get it.
Mrs. Baker:	Thanks.

(After 10 minutes, Mrs. Baker follows Nurse Jackie back to Dr. Green's Office.)

Dr. Green:	Mrs. Baker, your urine pregnancy test is positive.
Mrs. Baker:	Which means?
Dr. Green:	Which means you are pregnant?
Mrs. Baker:	Really? Oh, my god! That's wonderful! My husband and I have been waiting for this for such a long time!
Dr. Green:	Congratulations!
Mrs. Baker:	Thank you so much! And do you think I should 5. _____ with you for the follow-up examinations?
Dr. Green:	Yes, you should. You are supposed to see me at 8-10 weeks after your last period, for your first prenatal visit. Let's see, probably that will be around the New Year. Jackie will help you with it and she will tell you how often you need to see me for the follow-up visits. OK?
Mrs. Baker:	Sure! Thanks again! See you next time, bye!
Dr. Green:	You are welcome! Take care! Bye!

(373 words)

Comprehension of the text

Directions: *Please answer the questions according to the information from the dialogue.*

1. Why does Mrs. Baker go to see Dr. Green?

笔记

2. Does Mrs. Baker have any signs of early pregnancy?

3. What test does Dr. Green order for Mrs. Baker to confirm her pregnancy?

4. How long does it take for a patient to get the urine pregnancy test result?

5. When will Mrs. Baker see Dr. Green for her first prenatal visit?

Part B

Words in Focus

contraception /ˌkɒntrə'sepʃn/	n.	避孕，节育
diaphragm /'daiəfræm/	n.	避孕环
condom /'kɒndəm/	n.	避孕套，保险套
calculate /'kælkjuleit/	vt.	计算
parturition /ˌpɑːtjʊ'riʃn/	n.	生产，分娩
delivery /di'livəri/	n.	分娩
caesarean /si'zeəriən/	n.	剖腹产，<医>剖腹产的
trimesters /trai'mestə(r)/	n.	三学期制，妊娠期
premature /'premətʃə(r)/	n.	早产儿
postmature /'pəʊstmətjʊə/	n.	过度成熟的（婴儿），过期产
stillborn /'stilbɔːn/	adj.	死产的，夭折的，流产的
miscarriage /'miskæridʒ/	n.	流产，早产
terminate /'tɜːmineit/	v.	结束；使终结
induce /in'djuːs/	v.	<医>诱导；引起
labour /'leibə/	n.	分娩
oxytocin /ˌɒksi'təʊsin/	n.	催产素
Contraction /kən'trækʃ(ə)n/	n.	子宫收缩

ER-9-5
扫一扫 读一读

ER-9-6
扫一扫 看一看

Useful Expressions

oral contraceptive pill	口服避孕药
intrauterine device (IUD)	宫内节育器
copper coil	（避孕）铜环
the expected date of delivery	预产期
last menstrual period (LMP)	末次月经
a spontaneous vaginal delivery(SVD)	自然分娩
delivered by caesarean section	经剖腹产取出
a full-term pregnancy	足月妊娠
umbilical cord	脐带
spontaneous abortion	自然流产
termination of pregnancy	终止妊娠
amniotic fluid	羊水

Text

Directions: *You're going to hear a short passage. Before listening, you will have 5 seconds to read each of the questions which accompany it. Listen to the passage and complete the sentences according to the information from the text.*

Background:

　　The following passage is about the definition and the basic information of contraception,

 笔记

129

ER-9-7
扫一扫 听一
听

ER-9-8
扫一扫 知情
节

labor and childbirth.

Comprehension of the text

Complete the sentences according to the information from the text.

1. Childbirth is also referred to by doctors as _____.

2. A baby that is born a week before the EDD is _____.

3. A _____ of pregnancy may be necessary for medical reasons.

4. A full-term pregnancy is _____ weeks, divided into _____ trimesters.

5. A _____ is another term for a spontaneous abortion.

Part Ⅱ　Speaking

This section is designed to test your speaking ability. After learning the following conversation A and B you will have some abilities of speaking skill in medical and nursing working and try to do the following speaking tasks.

Conversation 1

Antenatal Education

In a women's centre, RN Jackie is teaching expectant mother Mrs. Baker on how to take care of her and her baby while she's pregnant.

Nurse Jackie:　　Hello, Mrs. Baker! How are you doing?

Mrs. Baker:　　Hi! Jackie, I'm great!

Nurse Jackie:　　You are at 6 weeks gestation, right?

ER-9-9
扫一扫 听一
听

ER-9-10
扫一扫 知情
节

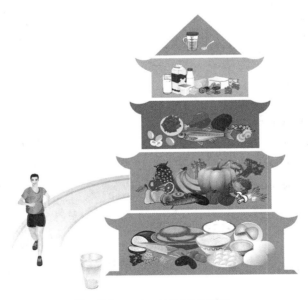

Fig. 9-1　antenatal education

Mrs. Baker:　　Correct.

Nurse Jackie:　　Then it's time for you to take prenatal education lessons.

Mrs. Baker:　　Is prenatal education very important?

Nurse Jackie:　　Yes. Prenatal care is very important. To help make sure that you and your baby

笔记

will be as healthy as possible, follow some simple guidelines and check in regularly with your doctor.

Mrs. Baker: OK. What will happen during prenatal visits?

Nurse Jackie: After you find out you are pregnant, you should make an appointment with your doctor. Your first prenatal visit will likely be when you are 6 to 8 weeks pregnant. Your doctor will probably start by talking to you about your medical history and how you've been feeling. You'll be weighed and have your blood pressure taken. These measurements will most likely be taken during each doctor's visit.

On your first visit, you'll also have a pelvic exam to check the size and shape of your uterus (womb) and a Pap smear to check for abnormalities of the cervix (the opening of the uterus).

Urine and blood tests samples will be taken on the first visit and again at later visits. Sometimes, an ultrasound may be done to help figure out when your baby is due or to check on your baby's growth and position in your uterus.

Mrs. Baker: Thank you, Jackie! How much weight should I gain during pregnancy?

Nurse Jackie: It's different for everyone, but most women gain about 25 to 30 pounds. If you don't weigh enough when you get pregnant, you may need to gain more. If you're overweight when you get pregnant, you may need to gain less.

Expectant Mother's Nutritional Needs

Nurse Jackie: Did you eat well last week?

Mrs. Baker: I didn't have a good appetite last week. I didn't want to eat. I'm wondering what should I eat?

Nurse Jackie: Eating a balanced diet is one of the most important things you can do for yourself and your baby. Well, the notion of "eating for two" may actually cause you to overestimate the amount of food you should eat during pregnancy.

Mrs. Baker: Overestimate? You mean I don't have to push myself to eat a lot?

Nurse Jackie: Exactly. Especially during the first trimester, the baby is still small, and you don't have to eat too much. A regular healthy woman usually has enough calories stored in her body for the baby to grow normally during the first trimester.

Mrs. Baker: It sounds like you don't suggest pregnant women push themselves to eat a lot, but how about in the 2nd or 3rd trimester? Should I push myself to eat more?

Nurse Jackie: In the 2nd and 3rd trimesters, a pregnant woman needs an additional 300 calories every day, and the most effective way to get the additional 300 calories is not pushing yourself to eat a lot, but by choosing the right food to eat.

Mrs. Baker: Well, what should I choose to eat, then?

Nurse Jackie: Here you go! I have a brochure with information about the Food Guide Pyramid. Why don't you take it and read it by yourself.

Mrs. Baker: What's the Food Guide Pyramid?

Nurse Jackie: The Food Guide Pyramid is designed to represent the food groups needed for a

笔记

balanced diet. Here, look at the picture, it's like a pyramid.

Mrs. Baker: OK, I will. And should I take vitamins?

Nurse Jackie: You should take 1,000 mcg (1 mg) of folic acid every day during your pregnancy. Folic acid can help prevent problems with your baby's brain and spinal cord. It is best to start taking folic acid before you get pregnant. Your doctor might want you to take a prenatal vitamin. If you do take a prenatal supplement, make sure you're not taking any other vitamin or mineral supplement along with it unless your doctor recommends it.

Mrs. Baker: It's really good to know. Thank you, Jackie!

Nurse Jackie: My pleasure, Mrs. Baker. There are a few foods that you should be more careful about eating while you are pregnant. Meat, eggs and fish that are not fully cooked could put you at risk for an infection. Remember to wash all fruit and vegetables. Keep cutting boards and dishes clean. Eat 4 or more servings of dairy foods each day. This will give you enough calcium for you and your baby. If you drink coffee or other drinks with caffeine, do not have more than 1 or 2 cups each day.

Mrs. Baker: OK! Thank you very much for all the information.

(806 words)

Words in Focus

gestation /dʒeˈsteɪʃn/	n.	怀孕；怀孕期
uterus /ˈjuː.tərəs/	n.	子宫
womb /wuːm/	n.	子宫
abnormality /ˌæbnɔːˈmæliti/	n.	畸形；反常，紊乱
cervix /ˈsɜːviks/	n.	颈部；子宫颈
preeclampsia /ˌpriːiˈklæmpsiːə/	n.	先兆子痫
syphilis /ˈsifilis/	n.	梅毒
overestimate /ˌəuvərˈestimeit/	vt.	对（数量）估计过高
calorie /ˈkæləri/	n.	卡路里；大卡
brochure /ˈbrəuʃ ə(r)/	n.	小册子，手册
infection /inˈfekʃn/	n.	<医>传染，感染
caffeine /ˈkæfiːn/	n.	咖啡碱；咖啡因；茶精

Useful Expressions

prenatal education	产前教育
a pelvic exam	骨盆检查
a Pap smear	一个子宫颈抹片检查
a balanced diet	均衡饮食
the Food Guide Pyramid	饮食指南金字塔

I. Free talk

Directions: *Work in pairs and discuss the following questions after learning to the recording of Dialogue One.*

1. What suggestions does nurse Jackie give to Mrs. Baker in terms of being pregnant?

_____

_____

ER-9-11
扫一扫 读一读

ER-9-12
扫一扫 看一看

笔记

2. What is the Food Guide Pyramid?

_____

_____

II. Comprehension of the text

Directions: *Fill in the blanks with the correct words given in the box.*

gestation	a balanced diet	infection	a Pap smear
the Food Guide Pyramid			

ER-9-13
扫一扫 答案
"晓"

1. Exactly which bacteria cause the _____ is still unknown.
2. You should get sufficient rest, eat _____, and exercise regularly.
3. Elephants have a _____ period of about 624 days.
4. He says most women diagnosed with cervical cancer in the United States have not had _____ in the three to five years prior to diagnosis.
5. _____ is a useful practical guide for attaining a balanced diet.

Conversation 2

Ending a Pregnancy(Abortion)

    Doctor Green is talking to students Amy and Betty about the basic knowledge of abortion—its definition, its 2 types and their procedures.

ER-9-14
扫一扫 听一
听

Doctor Green: Today, let's talk about abortion. What have you known about abortion?

Student Amy: Abortion means ending a pregnancy early.

Doctor Green: Yes. In some cases, a woman's pregnancy ends on its own. This is called a miscarriage, or a spontaneous abortion.

Student Betty: In other cases, a woman chooses to end her pregnancy by taking medicine (called medical abortion) or having surgery (called surgical abortion).

ER-9-15
扫一扫 知情
节

Doctor Green: Remember, these 2 types of abortion are usually done in the first trimester (the first 3 months) of the pregnancy.

Student Amy: And they are performed by a doctor and other health care professionals in the hospital, doctor's office or health center.

Doctor Green: Absolutely right!

Student Betty: It's dangerous to do a medical abortion in those illegal clinics.

Doctor Green: Yes. And what is a medical abortion then?

Student Betty: A medical abortion is an abortion caused by medicine.

Doctor Green: It can only be done in the first 9 weeks of pregnancy. What medicine does the most common type of medical abortion use?

Student Amy: It is called mifepristone. This is a pill that blocks progesterone, a hormone needed for pregnancy. It causes the lining of the womb (uterus) to become thin.

Doctor Green: For this procedure, a woman visits her doctor 3 times.

Student Betty: The woman takes mifepristone during the first visit, right?

Doctor Green: Yes, you are right. She comes back a few days later to take another medicine called misoprostol. Misoprostol makes the uterus contract and empty. Many women have been bleeding for about 13 days after taking

笔记

misoprostol. Light bleeding or discharge (called spotting) can continue for several weeks.

Student Amy: When do they do the last visit?

Doctor Green: After a couple of weeks, the woman will return to the doctor for a follow-up visit to be sure that the medicine was effective.

Student Amy: What does medical abortion feel like? Excuse my curiosity.

Doctor Green: For most women, medical abortion feels like a bad menstrual period with strong cramps, diarrhea and upset stomach. These symptoms are normal.

Student Betty: I'm wondering how effective a medical abortion is?

Doctor Green: Mifepristone is about 97% effective. In rare cases when medical abortion doesn't work, surgical abortion may be tried.

Student Betty: Then what is a surgical abortion?

Doctor Green: Surgical abortion is a procedure done by a doctor to remove the lining of the womb. There are 2 common procedures: manual vacuum aspiration (MVA), and dilatation and evacuation (D&E). They both use suction to empty the womb. MVA uses a handheld tool. D&E is done with a suction machine and tools.

MVA can be done in the first 12 weeks of pregnancy. D&E can be done after the first month of pregnancy and before the end of the 13th week.

Student Amy: Do we use any medicine for both procedures?

Doctor Green: Definitely! For both procedures, medicine can be given to help the woman feel calm. Then the doctor injects around the opening to the womb (called the cervix) with medicine to make it numb. The cervix is stretched open with a tool called a dilator, and the doctor inserts a tube. The uterus is emptied through this tube.

Student Betty: Excuse me. What does a surgical abortion feel like?

Doctor Green: For most women, surgical abortion feels like strong menstrual cramps. Women are usually given medicine to help with the pain and told to rest when they get home. Acetaminophen or ibuprofen can also help. Bleeding may continue off and on for a few weeks.

Student Betty: How effective is a surgical abortion?

Doctor Green: It is nearly 100% effective.

Student Amy: Many women may wonder if abortion would reduce their ability to get pregnant in the future?

Doctor Green: When done by health care professionals during the first trimester, both medical and surgical abortions are generally very safe. Serious complications are rare. Abortion generally does not reduce a woman's ability to get pregnant in the future.

(691 words)

Words in Focus

miscarriage /'miskærɪdʒ/	*n.*	流产，早产
discharge /dis'tʃɑːdʒ/	*n.*	流出；排放出的物体

笔记

mifepristone /mifipris'təʊn/	n.	米非司酮（一种堕胎药）
misoprostol /misɒp'rɒztl/	n.	米索前列醇
cramps /kræmps/	n.	痛性痉挛，抽筋
Acetaminophen /ə,si:tə'minəfen/	n.	扑热息痛；对乙酰氨基酚
ibuprofen /,aibju:'prəʊfen/	n.	布洛芬，异丁苯丙酸
procedure /prə'si:dʒə(r)/	n.	程序，过程，步骤
suction /'sʌkʃn/	n.	吸，抽吸
remove /ri'mu:v/	vt.	去除
insert /in'sɜːt/	vt.	插入；嵌入
stretch /stretʃ/	v.	伸展；延伸
dilator /dai'leitə/	n.	（外科用的）扩张器
numb /nʌm/	adj.	麻木的，失去感觉的

ER-9-16
扫一扫 读一读

ER-9-17
扫一扫 看一看

Useful Expressions

a spontaneous abortion	自然流产
medical abortion	药物流产
surgical abortion	人工流产术
health care professionals	医护人员
sanitary pads	卫生巾
manual vacuum aspiration	人工真空抽吸
dilatation and evacuation	扩张宫颈和清宫术

I. Match

Directions: Work in pairs read and recite the following dialogue.

A gynaecologist is talking to a 30-year-old woman.

Gynaecologist	Patient
Are Your periods regular?	Yes.
How often do you get them?	Every four weeks.
How old were you when you started to get them?	About 12.
When was your last period?	A week ago.
How long do the periods last usually?	4 or 5 days.
Would you say they are light or heavy?	Light.
Do you get clots?	No.
Do you get period pains?	Not really.
Is there any discharge between the periods?	A little.
What colour is it?	White.

II. Comprehension of the text

Directions: According to the following conversation and complete the sentences.

Miscarriage	procedure	stretch	off and on
health care professionals			

ER-9-18
扫一扫 答案
"晓"

1. It has been drizzling _____ for days.

2. Through the selfless and dedicated efforts of _____, the Hospital Authority has indeed

笔记

135

provided quality patient care to meet the needs of the community as a whole.

3. The ＿＿＿＿＿ of our plans was a great blow.

4. What's the ＿＿＿＿＿ for opening a savings account?

5. The exercises are designed to stretch and tone your leg muscles.

Part Ⅲ　Reading

Text A

ER-9-19
扫一扫 听一
听

ER-9-20
扫一扫 知情
节

> PIH is a common complication of pregnancy. This passage is about its serious consequences, the different types of PIH and who is at high risk of PIH.
>
> ***Pre-reading***
>
> 1. What is blood pressure?
> 2. What is PIH?
> 3. What are the different types of high blood pressure during pregnancy?

Pregnancy-induced Hypertension Syndrome (PIH)

Introduction

Hypertension is a common complication of pregnancy that may have serious consequences to the mother and fetus. The rising incidence of the disease reaches to 9.4% of pregnancies in China and 7% to 12% in other countries. PIH is one of the main causes of maternal and postnatal morbidity and mortality.

Who is at risk for PIH?

PIH is more common during a woman's first pregnancy and in women whose mothers or sisters had PIH. The risk of PIH is higher in women carrying multiple babies, in teenage mothers and in women older than 40 years of age. Other women at risk include those who had high blood pressure or kidney disease before they became pregnant.

What are the different types of high blood pressure during pregnancy?

There are three types of high blood pressure in pregnant women:

- **Chronic hypertension:** High blood pressure that develops before the 20th week of pregnancy or is present before the woman becomes pregnant. Sometimes a woman has high blood pressure for a long time before she gets pregnant, but she doesn't know it until her first prenatal check-up.

- **Gestational hypertension:** Some women just get high blood pressure near the end of pregnancy. They don't have any other associated symptoms.

- **Pregnancy-induced hypertension (PIH),** also called toxemia or preeclampsia: This condition can cause serious problems for both the mother and the baby if left untreated. PIH develops after the 20th weeks of pregnancy. Along with high blood pressure, it causes protein in the urine, blood changes and other problems.

What are the risks of PIH to the baby and me?

PIH can prevent the placenta (which gives oxygen and food to your baby) from getting

笔记

enough blood. If the placenta doesn't get enough blood, your baby gets less oxygen and food. This can cause low birth weight and other problems for the baby.

Most women who have PIH still deliver healthy babies. A few develop a condition called eclampsia (PIH with seizures), which is very serious for the mother and baby, or other serious problems. Fortunately, PIH is usually detected early in women who get regular prenatal care, and most problems can be prevented.

(367 words)

Words in Focus

maternal /məˈtɜːn(ə)l/	*adj.*	母亲的
postnatal /pəʊstˈneitl/	*adj.*	出生后的
morbidity /mɔːˈbidəti/	*n.*	发病率
placenta /pləˈsentə/	*n.*	胎盘
toxemia /tɒksˈiːmiə/	*n.*	毒血症；血毒症
eclampsia /ɪˈklæmpsiə/	*n.*	子痫；惊厥
detect /diˈtekt/	*vt.*	查明

ER-9-21
扫一扫 读一读

Useful Expressions

blood vessels	血管
chronic hypertension	慢性高血压
gestational hypertension	妊娠高血压
pregnancy-induced hypertension	妊高征

ER-9-22
扫一扫 看一看

Post-reading

I. Check your vocabulary

Find a word or phrase from the box below to complete each sentence.

protein	seizure	oxygen	detect	symptoms

1. The brain requires a constant supply of _____ .

2. He's complaining of all the usual flu _____ -a high temperature, headache and so on.

3. Peas and beans are a good source of vegetable _____ .

4. He had a _____ , and her heart stopped.

5. High levels of lead were _____ in the atmosphere.

ER-9-23
扫一扫 答案 "晓"

II. Check your comprehension

Read the following statements and then decide whether each of them is true or false based on the information from the text. Write T for true and F for false in the space provided.

(　　) 1. PIH is the main causes of maternal and postnatal morbidity and mortality.

(　　) 2. Those women who had high blood pressure before they became pregnant are at a higher risk of PIH.

(　　) 3. There are three types of PIH: chronic hypertension, gestational hypertension and preeclampsia.

(　　) 4. PIH develops after the 10th weeks of pregnancy.

(　　) 5. Women who have PIH can't deliver healthy babies.

ER-9-24
扫一扫 练一练

笔记

III. Supplementary

Text B

ER-9-25
扫一扫 听一
听

ER-9-26
扫一扫 知情
节

Worldwide, cervical cancer is the third most common cancer in women. In this text, you will learn something about its definition, Pap smear test and risk factors.

Pre-reading

1. What are the common Gynecological Cancers?
2. What is Cervical Cancer?
3. What is a Pap smear?

Cervical Cancer

Introduction (Incidence and Prevalence)

Worldwide, cervical cancer is the third most common cancer in women.

The incidence of cervical cancer in many countries has decreased greatly since the introduction of a screening program for detecting precancerous cervical intraepithelial neoplasia.

Definition

Cervical cancer is a malignant neoplasm arising from the uterine cervix.

What is a Pap smear?

A Pap smear is a test your doctor does to check for signs of cancer of the cervix.The cells from your cervix are checked for signs that they're changing from normal cells to abnormal cells. Before they turn into cancer, cells go through a series of changes. The results of your Pap smear can show whether your cells are going through these changes long before you actually have cancer. If caught and treated early, cervical cancer is not life threatening. This is why it is so important that you get regular Pap smears.

What happens during a Pap smear?

During a Pap smear, your doctor will put a special instrument called a speculum into your vagina. This helps open your vagina so the doctor can see your cervix and take a sample. Your doctor will gently clean your cervix with a cotton swab and then collect a sample of cells with a small brush, a tiny spatula or a cotton swab. Your doctor will put this sample on a glass slide and send it to a lab to be checked under a microscope.

What do the results mean?

A normal Pap smear means that all the cells in your cervix are normal and healthy. An abnormal Pap smear can be a sign of a number of changes in the cells on your cervix, including:

Inflammation (irritation).

This can be caused by an infection of the cervix, including a yeast infection, infection with the human papillomavirus (HPV), the herpes virus, or many other infections.

Abnormal cells.

These changes are called cervical dysplasia. The cells are not cancer cells, but may be precancerous (which means they could eventually turn into cancer).

More serious signs of cancer.

These changes affect the top layers of the cervix but don't go beyond the cervix.

More advanced cancer.

笔记

138

If the results of your Pap smear are abnormal, your doctor may want to do another Pap smear or may want you to have a colposcopy. A colposcopy gives your doctor a better look at your cervix and allows him or her to take a sample of tissue (called a biopsy).

How often should I have a Pap smear?

Every 3 years beginning at 21 years of age and continuing until 65 years of age.

If you're older than 65 years of age, talk with your doctor about how often you need a Pap smear. If you've been having Pap smears regularly and they've been normal, you may not need to keep having them.

How reliable is the test?

No test is perfect, but the Pap smear is a reliable test. It has helped drastically lower the number of women who die of cervical cancer.

Risk factors for cervical cancer

The main risk factors for cervical cancer are related to sexual practices. Risk factors for cervical cancer include sexual intercourse at an early age, multiple sex partners, tobacco smoking, long-term oral contraceptive use, low socioeconomic status, immunosuppressive therapy, and micronutrient deficiency.

Is there anything I can do to avoid getting cervical cancer?

You may be able to reduce your risk of cervical cancer if you: Delay sexual intercourse until you're 18 years of age or older. Make sure both you and your partner are tested for sexually transmitted infection (STIs).Limit your number of sex partners. Always use latex condoms to protect against STIs. (Remember condoms aren't 100% effective.)Avoid smoking.

(623 words)

Words in Focus

abnormal /æbˈnɔːml/	*adj.*	反常的，异常的
prevalence /ˈprevələns/	*n.*	（疾病等的）流行程度
precancerous /priːˈkænsərəs/	*adj.*	癌症前期的
reliable /rɪˈlaɪəbl/	*adj.*	可靠的
irritation /ˌɪrɪˈteɪʃn/	*n.*	刺激
papillomavirus /ˌpæpiˈləuməˈvaɪərəs/	*n.*	乳头瘤病毒
colposcopy /ˈkɒlpɒskəpi/	*n.*	阴道镜；阴道窥器检查
eventually /iˈventʃuəli/	*adv.*	终究；终于，最后
speculum /ˈspekjələm/	*n.*	金属镜，诊视器
drastically /ˈdræstikəli/	*adv.*	大大地，彻底地
screening /ˈskriːniŋ/	*n.*	筛查

Useful Expressions

Cervical cancer	宫颈癌
cervical intraepithelial neoplasia	宫颈上皮内瘤变
a cotton swab	棉拭子
cervical dysplasia	宫颈非典型增生
precancerous lesion	癌前病变
sexually transmitted infection	性传播感染
latex condom	乳胶避孕套
sexual intercourse	性交

ER-9-27
扫一扫 读一读

ER-9-28
扫一扫 看一看

笔记

Post-reading

I. Check your comprehension

Read the following statements and then decide whether each of them is true or false based on the information from the text. Write T for true and F for false in the space provided.

(   ) 1. A Pap smear is a test your doctor does to check for signs of cancer.

(   ) 2. The results of your Pap smear can show whether your cells are going through these changes long before you actually have cancer.

(   ) 3. Cervical cancer is life threatening and there is no cure at all.

(   ) 4. Having had many sexual partners may put you at risk for cervical cancer.

(   ) 5. Having Pap smears regularly can be helpful to lower the number of people who die of cervical cancer.

II. Discussing

Answer the following questions with the information from the text.

1. What is the incidence and prevalence of cervical cancer in most countries?

_____

_____

2. What is a Pap smear?

_____

_____

3. What happens during a Pap smear?

_____

_____

4. What is the main risk factor for cervical cancer?

_____

_____

5. What can we do to avoid getting cervical cancer?

_____

_____

III. Supplementary

ER-9-29
扫一扫 答案
"晓"

ER-9-30
扫一扫 练一
练

Part IV   Writing

Pregnancy Guidance for Women Who Have PIH

Instructions:

A woman who has been pregnant for 30 weeks and is considered at high risk for PIH. Please write a pregnancy guidance for her in English.

_____

_____

_____

_____

ER-9-31
扫一扫 答案
"晓"

笔记

Part V Enriching your word power

1. gynec(o)-; gynae-; gynaeco-; gyneco-; gyno-　　性，女子
   gynecogenic /gainekəudˈʒenik/　　女性化的
   gynecopathy /ˌdʒiniˈkɒpəθi/　　妇科病
2. perine(o)-　　会阴
   perineal /periˈniːəl/　　会阴的
   perineoplasty /periniːəuˈplæsti/　　会阴成形术
3. cervic(o)-　　颈
   cervicitis /ˌsɜːviˈsaitis/　　子宫颈炎
   cervicovaginitis /sɜːviˈkʌvidʒinaitəs/　　子宫颈阴道炎
4. colp(o)-; vagin(o)-　　阴道
   colporrhaphy /kɒlˈpɔːrəfi/　　阴道缝（合）术
   vaginodynia /ˈvædʒinɒdiniə/ 同 colpodynia　　阴道痛
5. hyster(o)-; metr(o)-; uter(o)-　　子宫
   hysterocarcinoma /histərəukɑːsiˈnəumə/　　子宫癌
   metrostenosis /metrɒsteˈnəusis/　　子宫狭窄
   uterotomy /ˈjuːtərɒtəmi/ 同 hysterotomy　　子宫切开术
6. mast(o)-; mamm(o)-　　乳房
   mastoptosis /mɑːsˈtɒptəusis/　　乳房下垂
   mammoplasty /ˈmæməplæsti/　　乳房成形术
7. men(o)-　　月经
   menopause /ˈmenəpɔːz/　　绝经期，更年期，活动终止期
   menolipsis /miˈnɒlipsis/　　停经；月经暂停
8. oophor(o)-; ovari(o)-　　卵巢
   oophoritis /ˌəuəfəˈraitis/　　卵巢炎
   ovariorrhexis /əuveəriɔːˈreksis/　　卵巢破裂
9. pelv(i)-　　骨盆
   pelvisection /pelviˈsekʃn/　　骨盆切开术
   pelvicellulitis /pelvaiseˈluːlitis/ 同 pelvic cellulitis　　盆腔蜂窝组织炎
10. ped(o)-　　儿童，足
    pediatrics /ˌpiːdiˈætriks/　　小儿科
    pedionalgia /piːdiəˈnældʒə/　　足底痛，跖痛
11. ante-; pre-; pro-　　（在）前
    anteflexed /æntfˈlekst/　　前屈的
    premature /ˈpremətʃə(r)/　　未成熟的，太早的，早熟的
    progeria /prəuˈdʒiəriə/　　早衰，早老儿童的早衰症
12. post-　　后
    postmenstrua /ˈpəustmenstrjuə/　　经后期
    postpuberal /pəustpˈjuːbrəl/　　青春期后的
13. neo-　　新
    neogenesis /ˌniːəuˈdʒenisis/　　再生，新生

笔记

neonate /'niːəʊneit/		（尤指出生不满一个月的）婴儿

14. placenta-　　　　　　　　　　　　　　　　　　　（胎盘）
　　placental /pləˈsentl/　　　　　　　　　　　　胎盘的
　　placenta praevia /pləˈsentə/　/pˈriːvaɪə/　　前置胎盘
　　abruptio placentae /æbˈrʌpʃɪəʊ/　/pləˈsentiː/　胎盘早剥

15. pre-(prae-)　　　　　　　　　　　　　　　　　前，前期
　　praevia /pˈriːvaiə/　　　　　　　　　　　　　前置的
　　preclinical /priˈklinikəl/　　　　　　　　　　临床前的
　　prelacteal /preˈlæktiəl/　　　　　　　　　　哺乳前的
　　premenopausal /pˈriːminəpɔːzl/　　　　　　绝经前期的
　　prenatal /ˌpriːˈneitl/　　　　　　　　　　　产前的
　　preoperative /priˈɒpərətiv/　　　　　　　　手术前的
　　prepuberty /priːˈpjuːbəti/　　　　　　　　　青春前期

16. post-　　　　　　　　　　　　　　　　　　　后，在后
　　postadolescence /pəʊstædəˈlesns/　　　　　壮年期
　　postdelivery /'pəʊst diˈlivəri/　　　　　　产后的
　　postnatal /'pəʊstˈneitl/　　　　　　　　　　产后的
　　postpartum /ˌpəʊstˈpɑːtəm/　　　　　　　　产后的
　　postmenopausal /'pəʊstmenəʊˈpɔːzəl/　　　绝经后的
　　postanesthesia /'pəʊst ˌænəsˈθiːziə/　　　麻醉后
　　postoperation /'pəʊst ˌɒpəˈreiʃn/　　　　手术后
　　postprandial /ˌpəʊstˈprændiəl/　　　　　　饭后的
　　posttraumatic /pəʊsttrɔːˈmætik/　　　　　创伤后的
　　postcoital /'pəʊstkɔitl/　　　　　　　　　性交后的

17. hyster-　　　　　　　　　　　　　　　　　　子宫
　　hysterectomy /ˌhistəˈrektəmi/　　　　　　子宫切除术
　　hysterocarcinoma /histərəʊkɑːsiˈnəʊmə/　子宫癌
　　hysteroscopy /histəˈrɒskəpi/　　　　　　　子宫镜检查
　　hysterospasm /histərəʊsˈpæzəm/　　　　　子宫痉挛

18. gyneco-　　　　　　　　　　　　　　　　　女性
　　gynecology /ˌgaɪniˈkɒlədʒi/　　　　　　　妇科学
　　gynecopathy /ˌdʒiniˈkɒpəθi/　　　　　　　妇科病
　　gynecology /ˌgaɪniˈkɒlədʒi/　　　　　　　妇科
　　gynecologist /ˌgaɪniˈkɒlədʒist/　　　　　妇科医生

19. 相关词汇
　　uterus /'juːtərəs/　　　　　　　　　　　　子宫
　　cervix /'sɜːviks/　　　　　　　　　　　　　子宫颈
　　fundus /'fʌndəs/　　　　　　　　　　　　　底
　　pregnancy /'pregnənsi/　　　　　　　　　怀孕
　　delivery /dɪˈlivəri/（labor，childbirth）　　分娩
　　amnion /'æmniən/　　　　　　　　　　　　羊膜
　　corpus /'kɔːpəs/　　　　　　　　　　　　　白体
　　corpus luteum /'kɔːpəs/　/'luːtiːəm/　　　黄体

menstruation /ˌmenstruˈeiʃn/   月经

umbilical cord /ʌmˌbilikl ˈkɔːd/   脐带

embryo /ˈembriəu/   胚胎

amniotic fluid /ˌæmniɒtik ˈfluːid/   羊水

pap smear /pæp smiə/   巴氏涂片；（子宫抹片）

cervical biopsy /ˈsəːvikəl baiˈɔpsi/   宫颈活检

fallopian tube /fəˈlɒpeən/ /tjuːb/   输卵管

ovary /ˈəuvəri/   卵巢

ovum /ˈəuvəm/   卵子

perineum /ˌperiˈniːəm/   会阴

vagina /vəˈdʒainə/   阴道

vulva /ˈvʌlvə/   外阴

labia /ˈleibiə/   阴唇

mons pubis /ˌmɒnz ˈpjuːbis/   阴阜

hymen /ˈhaimən/   处女膜

birth control /bəːθ kənˈtrəul/   节育

umbilical cord /ʌmˌbilikl ˈkɔːd/   脐带

breast-feeding /brest ˈfiːdiŋ/   母乳喂养

Part Ⅵ Exercise

Directions: *In this section, only one of the following options is correct, please choose.*

（封育新　吕小君）

ER-9-32
扫一扫 看一看

笔记

Unit 10
Pediatric Department

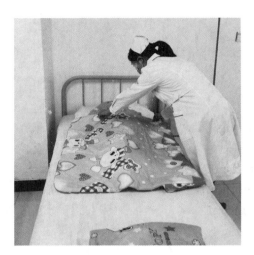

Fig. 10-1   pediatric ward

Early to bed and early to rise, makes a man healthy, wealthy and wise.

早睡早起会使人健康、富有和聪明。

——Benjamin Franklin（本杰明·富兰克林）

Learning Objectives

Skill focus

1. *Master the examination of the child undergoing cardiac catheterization, the nursing of the child with pneumonia and diarrhea, the writing of birth certificate.*

2. *Know the different symptoms, complications, treatments and nursing between measles and chickenpox.*

3. *Understand something about sickle cell anemia.*

Language focus

1. *Have ability of talking with the patient's relatives and relieving their anxiety.*

2. *Have ability of creating and guessing a new word using roots, prefix or suffix.*

Part I   Listening

This section is designed to test your ability to understand spoken English in nursing or medical contexts. You will hear a selection of recorded materials and you must answer the questions that accompany them. There are TWO parts in this section, Part A and Part B.

Part A

Words in Focus

catheterization /kæθitərai'zeiʃən/	*n.*	插管术；导尿术
prior /'praiə(r)/	*adj.*	在……之前；优先的
attach /ə'tætʃ/	*v.*	把……固定；附上，系
neonate /'ni:əuneit/	*n.*	新生儿
umbilical /ʌm'bilikəl/	*adj.*	脐带的；母系的
approach /ə'prəutʃ/	*n.*	方法；途径；接近
caution /'kɔ:ʃn/	*v.*	警告；提醒
perform /pə'fɔ:m/	*v.*	执行；完成；做；运行

ER-10-1
扫一扫 读一读

ER-10-2
扫一扫 看一看

Useful Expressions

take hypersensitive test	皮试
pass through	经过；通过

Text

Directions: *In this section you will hear a short passage, at the end of the passage, one or more questions will be asked about what was said, decide which the best answer is.*

Background:

The following passage is about cardiac catheterization, which will introduce what it is, what we should do before it, and what we ought to do during the procedure.

ER-10-3
扫一扫 听一听

Comprehension of the Text

1. Where does the radiopaque catheter pass through?

   A. a vein in the arm   B. an artery in the neck   C. leg

2. Which needn't be prepared before the operation?

   A. clean or shave the area of skin

   B. check blood type and prepare blood

   C. assess pulse, blood pressure, and respirations frequently

3. In the cardiac catheterization room, how to insert the catheter into the right side of the heart?

   A. through an umbilical artery

   B. an arterial approach

   C. a venous approach

ER-10-4
扫一扫 知情节

4. According to the passage, which of the following statements is true?

   A. When insert the catheter, their heart may momentarily speed up.

   B. When insert the catheter, they will feel nothing.

   C. When insert the catheter, they will hurt.

5. Why must the light be turned off when the medicine is injected?

   A. Because the children need sleep.

   B. Because the doctor can watch the medicine on a television screen as it passes through the heart.

   C. Because it is daytime.

Part B

Words in Focus

relatively /'relətɪvli/	*adv.*	相对地；比较地

笔记

ER-10-5
扫一扫 读一读

ER-10-6
扫一扫 看一看

ER-10-7
扫一扫 听一听

ER-10-8
扫一扫 知情节

support /sə'pɔːt/	v.	支持；支撑；维持
clinical /'klinikl/	adj.	临床的；诊所的
defect /'diːfekt/	n.	毛病；欠缺，缺点
trauma /'trɔːmə/	n.	损伤；创伤；挫折
inhalation /ˌinhə'leiʃn/	n.	吸入；吸入剂，吸入物

Useful Expressions

be related to	与……有关；与……有联系
suffer from	患（某种病）；遭受折磨

Text

Directions: *You're going to hear one conversation. Before listening, you will have 5 seconds to read each of the questions which accompany it. Listen to the passage and answer the following questions.*

Background:

The following conversation is between the patient's mother and the nurse. The patient's name is Feng Feng. He is a child with a congenital heart disease and infection. The child is having a fever and the child's mother worries. The nurse explains and comforts her patiently.

Comprehension of the text

1. What's wrong with Feng *Feng*?

_____

_____

2. How to treat the patient's bronchopneumonia?

_____

_____

3. Are there any methods of curing the baby's heart disease?

_____

_____

4. What's the better treatment for the patient's heart disease?

_____

_____

5. Do you think the nurse is qualified? Why?

_____

_____

Part II   Speaking

This section is designed to test your speaking ability. After learning the following conversation A and B you will have the ability of speaking skill in nursing the children with pneumonia and diarrhea, and try to do the following speaking tasks.

Conversation 1

Educating a Relative of a Patient with Pneumonia

Dou Dou is a two-year-old boy. He has been in hospital for pneumonia for five days. Mrs. Li is his mother. She feels worried because her baby still has a fever and coughs badly. What's

笔记

more, the doctor advised Mrs. Li do the nebulization for her baby, she asks the nurse something about it. The nurse explains to her how to relieve the child's symptoms and comforts her.

Nurse: Mrs. Li, is your baby getting any better?

Mrs. Li: He seems to be getting worse. He had the intravenous transfusion for 3～4 days without any improvement. When he coughs, there's something in his throat.

Nurse: How did the doctor say about the symptom?

Mrs. Li: The doctor advised if my baby coughs badly and wheezes, the nebulization can be done for him. Does it have side effects for children? Does he need to inhale every time he coughs?

Nurse: Don't feel too worried, Mrs. Li. The nebulization doesn't cause side effects, and your baby doesn't need the drug if he doesn't wheeze.

Mrs. Li: But he coughs so seriously!

Nurse: Some baby patients have a dry cough at the early stage of pneumonia. As time goes on, the dead bacteria and virus become sputum, which is a waste product that is being cleaned from the body's respiration system. There is a disease development process. You need not worry too much. We are giving the baby a very effective treatment, but it takes time for the drugs to take effects. Let's try to be more patient, OK?

Mrs. Li: We are very worried for our only baby since he has been ill for more than 10 days.

Nurse: I can understand how you feel. However, your worries can't solve any problems. Rather, it will affect your own immune system. You should take better care of yourself. Otherwise, you'll get sick, which in turn will affect your baby's health. So you should get more rest and eat more nutritious foods to increase your resistance to diseases.

Mrs. Li: Then what should I pay attention to?

Nurse: At home you should open the windows frequently to keep the air fresh. When your baby coughs, pat his back softly to help him cough up sputum. When patting, you should close your five fingers of your hand and pat on the baby's back with only the edge of the hand.

Demonstrated how to pat.

Nurse: What's more, your baby is too young to spit, so he can only swallow it. When you find some mucus in her stool, it's the sputum that he had swallowed.

Mrs. Li: Oh, now I see. I thought it was the bad food he ate.

Nurse: Sometimes because the sputum stimulates the gastrointestinal track or due to the virus's effect, some babies will have diarrhea.

Mrs. Li: It's terrible! What should we do?

Nurse: You needn't worry because not every baby has diarrhea. Since your baby has a fever, we'll take his temperature every 4 hours. Please call us to measure his temperature at any time if you feel he has a fever. If his temperature is too high, the doctor will give him an antipyretic. Please don't give him any medicine yourself. Feed your baby more water and change his clothes when he is perspiring too much. You may put a dry towel on his back to prevent him catching cold. I will come around some time later. You may press the call button to call us if you need us.

ER-10-9
扫一扫 听一听

ER-10-10
扫一扫 知情节

笔记

Mrs. Li: OK. Thank you!

Nurse: You are welcome. It's my job.

(470 words)

Words in Focus

ER-10-11
扫一扫 读一
读

improvement /im'pruːvmənt/	*n.*	改进，改善
nebulization /ˌnebjʊlaɪˈzeiʃən/	*n.*	喷雾疗法，喷雾作用
serious /'siəriəs/	*adj.*	严肃的，严重的；重要的
product /'prɒdʌkt/	*n.*	产品；结果
effective /iˈfektiv/	*adj.*	有效的；起作用的
resistance /riˈzistəns/	*n.*	抵抗；抗力
softly /'sɒftli/	*adv.*	柔和地；柔软地；温和地
prevent /priˈvent/	*v.*	预防；阻止；阻碍

ER-10-12
扫一扫 看一
看

Useful Expressions

intravenous transfusion	静脉输液
side effects	副作用
due to	由于，因为

I. Free talk

Directions: *Work in pairs and discuss the following questions after listening to the recording of Conversation One.*

1. Explain to your partner how to care for the children with pneumonia?

_____

_____

2. What is the matter with the patient?

_____

_____

II. Comprehension of the text

Directions: *Complete the sentences according to the conversation.*

1. If my baby coughs badly and _____, the nebulization can be done for him.

    A. has a sore throat   B. fever   C. wheezes

2. As time goes on, the disintegrated granulocytes and dead bacteria and virus become _____.

    A. saliva（唾液）   B. sputum   C. waste material

3. So you should _____ and eat more nutritious foods to increase your resistance to diseases.

    A. get more rest   B. drink some water   C. do some exercises

4. When your baby coughs, pat his _____ softly to help him cough up sputum.

    A. chest   B. back   C. neck

5. You may put _____ on his back to prevent him catching cold.

    A. clean clothes   B. a small blanket   C. a dry towel

III. Group work

    Work in pairs. If student A is a nurse and student B is a patient's mother. The child has been in hospital for pneumonia for several days, but he still has a fever. His mother is dissatisfied with the treatment. You may begin like this:

Student A: Good morning, Mrs. Chen. How is your baby?

笔记

Student B: What's the matter? Our child has been in hospital for two or three days. Why hasn't his fever gone down?

......

Conversation 2

Comforting a Relative of a Patient with Diarrhea

Mrs. Li is the patient's mother. Her baby is only ten-month-old. The baby suffers from diarrhea and has been admitted into hospital for 2 days. Because her baby's conditions haven't improved significantly, Mrs. Li distrusts the treatment. The nurse explains to her, comforts her patiently, and gives some humane care.

Nurse: Good afternoon, Mrs. Li. Does the baby have his bowels open a bit less today?

Mrs. Li: No, still a lot.

Nurse: Do you remember how many times he went toilet?

Mrs. Li: I can't remember exactly. It must have been over four times.

Nurse: What kind of stool did you notice, watery or mucous?

Mrs. Li: They are quite loose with milk curd and undigested food in them. Are the drugs you used for my child correct?

Nurse: We are responsible for every patient. There are certain principles to the treatment of every disease. The dosage of the drug was calculated according to the baby's age and the weight. Please don't worry.

Mrs. Li: How could I not worry! What I'm concerned about the most is that you might have delayed his treatment.

Nurse: I can understand how you feel. Please believe me because what I said to you was from my heart. People used to say "To recover from an illness is like reeling off raw silk from the cocoons". It will take certain process for the disease to become better. What your baby got is viral enteritis, and in general, is a virus infected disease which needs about one week or more to recover.

Mrs. Li: Look, the child has diarrhea again. Call the doctor quickly.

The baby is crying.

Nurse: OK, don't worry. I call the doctor right away.

            After examining the baby, the doctor thinks the water content in the stool has decreased, the illness has taken a favorable turn.

Mrs. Li: You keep saying the illness is getting better. I know you do not care about my child.

Nurse: The doctors here are very experienced. The doctor who examined your child also has tested the pH value of his excrement. The situation is really much better.

Mrs. Li prepares to change the diaper for the child.

Nurse: Mrs. Li, let me help you.

The nurse washed the buttock of the baby with warm water and put on a clean diaper.

Nurse: Mrs. Li, the baby's stool is much better. But he still should be fed with lactose free milk powder. It is easy to digest and is good for the intestines mucous membrane to repair. Also, your diet should be light at the present time, so that there will be less fat in your breast milk. In addition, you should give more water to the baby to supplement the baby's water need.

ER-10-13
扫一扫 答案
"晓"

ER-10-14
扫一扫 听一
听

ER-10-15
扫一扫 知情
节

笔记

Mrs. Li:　Your attitude is not too bad.

Nurse:　　Thank you. The baby is about to sleep. I will come to see him later.

Two hours later, the nurse came back a second time to his bedside.

Mrs. Li:　Thank you very much. My baby has not had a bowel movement for two hours. I feel much better now.

(468 words)

Words in Focus

ER-10-16
扫一扫 读一读

ER-10-17
扫一扫 看一看

defecate /ˈdefikeit/	v.	排便；澄清
dosage /ˈdəusidʒ/	n.	（药物等的）剂量；服法
delay /dɪˈlei/	v.	耽搁；延期；推迟
content /ˈkɔntent/	n.	内容；满足；容量
situation /ˌsitʃuˈeiʃn/	n.	情况；形势，处境
digest /daiˈdʒest/	v.	消化；吸收
supplement /ˈsʌplimənt/	v.	增补；补充
attitude /ˈætitjuːd/	n.	态度；看法
bowel /ˈbauəl/	n.	肠；同情心
movement /ˈmuːvmənt/	n.	运动；活动

Useful Expressions

according to	根据；按照
be concerned about	关心；挂念
used to	过去常常

I. Free talk

Directions: *Work in pairs and discuss the following questions after learning Conversation Two.*

1. What is the patient's stool like?

_____

_____

2. How does Mrs. Li think of the treatment at first?

_____

_____

3. What is the attitude of the nurse?

_____

_____

4. What should the child's mother do?

The child still should be fed with _____. Also, the mother's diet should be _____ at the present time, so that there will be less _____ in her breast milk. In addition, she should _____ to the baby to supplement the baby's water need.

II. Conversation

ER-10-18
扫一扫 答案
"晓"

Directions: *If you are a nurse to give a patient's mother some humane care, when she worries and complains, what should you talk with her?*

_____

_____

III. Practice

Directions: *Read and practice the conversations after the recording.*

笔记

Part Ⅲ   Reading

Text A

> Measles and chickenpox are all infectious diseases. Their early symptoms are similar. This passage is about their different aspects of the definition, symptoms, complications, treatments and nursing.
>
> **Pre-reading**
> 1. What are symptoms of measles and chickenpox?
> 2. How to nurse the children with measles?

Measles and Chickenpox

Measles is an acute respiratory infectious disease caused by measles virus. Its characteristics are that rash spreads all over the neck, face, trunk, arms and legs from first to last, accompanied by high fever. Chickenpox is a common acute infectious disease in childhood, which is caused by herpes virus.

The clinical symptoms of measles are different in three clinical stages, which are early period, eruption period, and recovery period. In early period, chief symptoms are similar to those of upper respiratory infection. Children have a high fever, headache, cough, sneeze, conjunctivitis, and tear. Koplic spots are favorable evidence for early diagnosis. The rash often appears after 3 or 4 days' fever. The rash usually starts along the hairline of the forehead, behind the ears, and spreads over the face, neck, trunk, entire arms and thighs, and finally, palms and soles within 2 or 3 days. It is red and irregular rash. The children feel itchy, but skin is normal. During this stage, children may appear very ill and may be delirious, have abdominal pain, diarrhea, and vomit. On the third or fourth day, the rash begins to fade in the same sequence in which it appears, followed with peeling and brown pigmentation. Its common complications are otitis media, pneumonia, and encephalitis.

The clinical symptoms of chickenpox are fever, discomfort, bad appetite, and slight abdominal pain. These appear in 24 to 48 hours before rash eruption. The spots of chickenpox start on scalp, face, and trunk. They are red and itching papules first, and then become clear and full blisters. After 3～4 days, the rash crusts rapidly. Chickenpox may be associated with several complications, including secondary infections of the lesions, pneumonia and encephalitis.

Measles needn't be treated by special antiviral therapy. The children should stay in bed and drink more boiled water. So when nursing the children with measles, the room should be ventilated twice a day. Clothes and quilts are proper, choosing the thin and soft clothing. Take bath and change clothes every day to keep skin clean and dry. Cut the child's fingernails short so that scratching will not open up lesions and cause secondary infection. Clean eyes with warm normal saline to remove secretions or crusts and use antibiotic drops or ointments. Keep vomitus and tears away from ears to avoid otitis media. Maintain respiratory tract clean. Be careful not to

ER-10-19
扫一扫 听一听

ER-10-20
扫一扫 知情节

笔记

low the temperature quickly for the child with a high fever.

　　Chickenpox can use antiviral treatment as early as possible. For the children with chickenpox, proper clothing and room temperature are needed to avoid irritable itching. Change clothes frequently and keep skin clean. Cut the child's fingernails short in order not to scratch the skin and cause secondary infection or scar. Bath the children with soda water to reduce the itch. Calamine lotion may be used too.

(477 words)

Words in Focus

ER-10-21
扫一扫 读一读

infectious /ɪnˈfekʃəs/	*adj.*	传染的；有传染性的
characteristics /ˌkærəktəˈrɪstɪks/	*n.*	特性，特征，特色
appear /əˈpɪə(r)/	*v.*	出现，显现
period /ˈpɪəriəd/	*n.*	时期；(一段)时间
evidence /ˈevɪdəns/	*n.*	证据；迹象；明显
irregular /ɪˈregjələ(r)/	*adj.*	不规则的；无规律的
itchy /ˈɪtʃi/	*adj.*	(使)发痒的
normal /ˈnɔːml/	*adj.*	正常的；标准的
antiviral /ˌæntiˈvaɪrəl/	*adj.*	抗病毒的
therapy /ˈθerəpi/	*n.*	治疗，疗法，疗效
ventilate /ˈventɪleɪt/	*v.*	通风；使通风
solution /səˈluːʃn/	*n.*	溶液；解决

ER-10-22
扫一扫 看一看

Useful Expressions

be similar to	与……相似
provide with	给……提供

Post-reading

I. Check your comprehension

Choose the best answer to complete each sentence with the information from the text.

1. Measles is an acute respiratory infectious disease caused by _____ virus.

　　A. herpes　　　　　　　B. measles　　　　　　　C. respiratory

2. In _____ period, chief symptoms of measles are similar to those of upper respiratory infection.

　　A. recovery　　　　　　B. eruption　　　　　　　C. early

3. _____ are favorable evidence for early diagnosis of measles.

　　A. Macula　　　　　　　B. papules　　　　　　　C. Koplic spots

4. The spots of chickenpox are itching red papules first, then become clear and full blisters.

　　A. Yes　　　　　　　　B. No　　　　　　　　　C. Not mentioned

5. Bath the children with _____ to reduce the itch.

　　A. soda water　　　　　B. saline water　　　　　C. alcohol

II. Check your vocabulary

Find a word or phrase from the box below to complete each sentence. Change word forms where necessary.

acute	characteristic	accompany	infectious	clinical
appear	complication	treat	solution	be similar to

1. Measles is an _____ respiratory infectious disease caused by measles virus.
2. Macula, papules, herpes, pustules, and crust appear at the same time in various stages is the _____ of chickenpox.
3. Rash spreads all over the neck, face, trunk, arms and legs from first to last, _____ by high fever.
4. Chickenpox is a common acute _____ disease in childhood.
5. The _____ symptoms of measles are different in three stages.
6. The rash _____ often after 3 or 4 days' fever.
7. Its common _____ are otitis media, pneumonia, encephalitis.
8. Measles needn't be _____ by special antiviral therapy.
9. Clean eyes with warm saline _____ to remove secretions or crusts.
10. In early period, chief symptoms _____ those of upper respiratory infection.

III. Supplementary

Text B

ER-10-23
扫一扫 答案
"晓"

> Sickle cell anemia is an inherited, lifelong disease, in which the patient's body produces abnormally shaped red blood cells. In this text, you will learn something about its symptoms, complications and treatment.
>
> ### Pre-reading
> 1. What is sickle cell anemia?
> 2. What are clinical symptoms of sickle cell anemia?

ER-10-24
扫一扫 练一练

Sickle Cell Anemia

Sickle cell anemia is an inherited, lifelong disease, in which the patient's body produces abnormally shaped red blood cells. The cells are shaped like a sickle. They don't last as long as normal and round red blood cells, which leads to anemia. Because of the defect of the hemoglobin, people with the disease are born with two sickle cell genes, one from each parent. If you only have one sickle cell gene, it's called sickle cell trait. About 1 in 12 African Americans has sickle cell trait. A blood test can show if you have the trait or anemia. In most states of America, the newborns will be examined through neonatal screening project for the diagnosis of sickle cell disease when they are at birth.

ER-10-25
扫一扫 听一听

ER-10-26
扫一扫 知情节

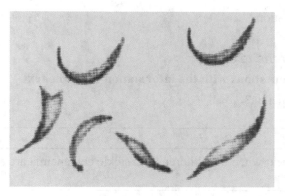

Fig. 10-2   sickle cell anemia

笔记

The clinical symptoms of sick newborns seldom appear, and hemolytic anemia will appear gradually. But the immune function of the infant with sickle cell anemia is abnormal. Many children are without functional spleen when they are at six months, which made bacterial sepsis become the most deadly danger. Acute sickle finger (toe) inflammation is often the first symptoms in children with sickle cell anemia. Acute painful blood vessel obstruction is the most prominent and common symptoms of sickle cell anemia. The other common symptoms include: anemia, abdominal pain, bone pain, breathlessness, delayed growth puberty, fatigue, fever, and jaundice.

Infection is a major complication of sickle cell anemia. Pneumonia is the leading cause of death in children with the condition. Other infections common in people with sickle cell anemia include meningitis, influenza, and hepatitis. If a child with sickle cell anemia shows early signs of an infection, such as fever, seek treatment right away. Another problem that must be paid attention to is to avoid dehydration. It is advised that the patient should drink at least 8 glasses of water every day, exercise regularly. But avoid overworking.

The most important part of the treatment is to prevent complications of sickle cell anemia and improve the health status of children. All the children with sickle cell anemia need to vaccinate with vaccines. The caregivers must be trained to know how to take body temperature accurately, assess diseases, touch spleen, and learn the symptoms of anemia and stroke. They also must know how to deal with pain and when need to go to the hospital. When treating acute chest syndrome and stroke, blood transfusion can be considered before operation. Bone marrow transplantation is the only way to cure sickle cell anemia, but It is only for children under 16 years of age and the patient must have the same cells with HLA(Human Leukocyte Antigen).

(442 words)

Words in Focus

inherit /inˈherit/	v.	继承；继任
abnormally /æbˈnɔːməli/	adv.	不正常地
trait /treit/	n.	过多，过量；超负荷
optimize /ˈɒptimaiz/	v.	使最优化，使尽可能有效
conventional /kənˈvenʃənl/	adj.	平常的；依照惯例的
syndrome /ˈsindrəʊm/	n.	综合症状；典型表现
cure /kjʊə(r)/	v.	治愈；矫正

Useful Expressions

lead to	导致；通往
bone marrow transplantation	骨髓移植

Post-reading

I. Comprehension of the text

Answer the following questions with the information from the text

1. What is sickle cell anemia?

_____

_____

2. What symptoms appear when the children with sickle cell anemia are at six months?

_____

_____

ER-10-27
扫一扫 读一读

ER-10-28
扫一扫 看一看

笔记

3. What is the most important part of the treatment?

_____

_____

4. Can all the children with sickle cell anemia be treated by bone marrow transplantation?

_____

_____

II. Vocabulary activities

Find a word or phrase from the box below to complete each sentence. Change word forms where necessary.

inherit	because of	trait	immune	inflammation
prominent	avoid	prevent	train	cure

1. Sickle cell anemia is an _____, lifelong disease.
2. _____ the defect of the hemoglobin molecule...
3. A blood test can show if you have the _____ or anemia.
4. But the _____ function of the infant with sickle cell anemia is abnormal.
5. Acute sickle finger (toe) _____ is often the first symptom in children with sickle cell aemia.
6. Acute painful blood vessel obstruction is the most _____ and common symptom of sickle cell anemia.
7. Another problem that must be paid attention to is to _____ dehydration.
8. The most important part of the treatment is to _____ complications of sickle cell anemia.
9. The caregivers must be trained to know how to take body temperature _____.
10. Bone marrow transplantation is the only way to _____ sickle cell anemia.

III. Supplementary

ER-10-29
扫一扫 答案
"晓"

ER-10-30
扫一扫 练一
练

Part Ⅳ　Writing

Writing a Birth Certificate

Instructions:

This article is about documentation relating to a baby's birth. A birth certificate is a statement issued by the hospital, which is used to prove when the baby was born, the baby's sex and birth place, who are parents and so on. It is a written material with a certain proving force and a long-term effect. And can be used as the basis for the baby registration account. It is a legal document to prove the origin of personal life.

Sentence Patterns:

中文证明书常以"兹证明……"开始，英语多译为"This is to certify that...".

A certificate usually consists of the following parts:

1. **the heading** (certificate)
2. **the body** (the main content of the certificate)
3. **the signature** (handwritten or typed)

笔记

Examples:

Birth Certificate

This is to certify that Tom Smith (male) was born on April 15, 2014 in Shanghai, China, to House Smith, father and Mary Smith, mother.

The City Hospital

(photo)　　　　　　　　　　　　　(sealed)

Signature:

(sealed)

Dated the 20th day of May,2014

Practice:

Write a birth certificate according to the following information.

姓名：李欣

性别：女

出生日期：2015 年 4 月 18 日

出生地：北京海淀区

父亲姓名：李磊

母亲姓名：孙薇

Birth Certificate

_____
_____
_____
_____
_____
_____
_____
_____
_____
_____
_____
_____

ER-10-31
扫一扫 答案
"晓"

Part Ⅴ　Enriching your word power

anterior fontanel /æn'tiəriːə ˌfɔntə'nel/	前囟门
posterior fontanel /pɔ'stiəriːə ˌfɔntə'nel/	后囟门
polio /'pəʊliəʊ/ 同 poliomyelitis	脊髓灰质炎；小儿麻痹症
myelitis /ˌmaiə'laitis/	脊髓炎
otitis externa /əʊ'taitis/ /ik'stɜːnl/	外耳炎
macrocephaly /mækrəʊ'səfəli/	巨头，巨头畸形
papule /'pæpjuːl/	丘疹
eczema /'eksimə/	湿疹
urticaria /ˌɜːti'keəriə/	荨麻疹
psoriasis /sə'raiəsis/	牛皮癣，银屑癣

笔记

omphalocele /ˈɒmfələʊsiːl/	脐突出
gastroschisis /ɡæsˈtrɒskisis/	腹裂（畸形）
dermatitis /ˌdɜːməˈtaitis/	皮炎
croup /kruːp/	义膜性喉炎
patent ductus arteriosus	动脉导管未闭
atrial septal defect(A.S.D.)	房间隔缺损
ventricular septal defect (V.S.D.)	室间隔缺损
tetralogy of fallot (T.O.F.)	法洛四联症
child Maltreatment (child abuse)	儿童虐待
attention deficit disorder (ADD)	儿童多动症
Sudden infant death syndrome(S.I.D.S.)	婴儿猝死综合征
Down's syndrome	唐氏综合征
cerebral palsy	脑瘫

Part Ⅵ　Exercise

Directions: *In this section, only one of the following options is correct, please choose.*

（陈明慧　吕小君）

ER-10-32
扫一扫 看一
看

笔记

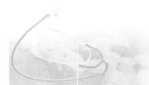

Unit 11
Geriatric Department

If there is one thing one can always yearn for and sometimes attain, it is human love.

如果有一件人可以永远渴望，而且有时能够得到的东西，那就是人类的爱。

——Albert Camus（阿尔贝·卡缪）

Learning Objectives

Skill focus

1. *Master the main symptoms of Alzheimer Disease and Depression, the musculoskeletal system of the elderly and guidelines of daily living about hip replacement.*

2. *Know some nursing interventions for the clients with Alzheimer Disease and depression.*

3. *Understand the falling of the elderly and promoting independence in the elderly.*

Language focus

1. *Describe the symptoms of Alzheimer Disease and depression with some medical terms.*

2. *Have ability of creating and guessing a new word using roots and prefix or suffix.*

Part I Listening

This section is designed to test your ability to understand spoken English in nursing or medical contexts. You will hear a selection of recorded materials and you must answer the questions that accompany them. There are TWO parts in this section, Part A and Part B.

Part A

Words in Focus

falling /ˈfɔːliŋ/	n.	落下，坠落
elderly /ˈeldəli/	n.	老年人
unintentional /ˌʌninˈtenʃənəl/	adj.	不是故意的；无意的，无心的
bifocal /ˌbaiˈfoukl/	n.	双光眼镜
severity /səˈvɛriti/	n.	严重，严重程度
deformity /diˈfɔːrməti/	n.	残缺，残废，畸形的人或物
compress /kəmˈprɛs/	vt.	压缩 / 敷布，压布
pedestrian /pəˈdɛstriən/	n.	步行者
fracture /ˈfræktʃə/	n.	破裂，骨折

Useful Expressions

personal injury	人身所受损害，人身伤害
risk factor	危险系数，危险因素

nursing home	小型私人医院；疗养院
road traffic accident	道路交通事故
health care	卫生保健

Text

Directions: In this section you will hear a short passage, at the end of the passage, one or more questions will be asked about what was said, decide which the best answer is.

Background:

　　Dr. Chad with his two students, Susanna and Helen, is talking about falling of the elderly.

Comprehension of the text

1. Falling is a major cause of _____, especially for the _____.

    A. property loss, young people

    B. losing their job, middle-aged people

    C. personal injury, elderly

2. Unintentional fallings resulted in 556,000 deaths in 2013 up from 341,000 deaths in 1990.

    A. yes   B. no   C. not mentioned

3. Even fallings from standing position to flat ground may cause serious injuries _____.

    A. in children   B. in elderly   C. in women

4. The severity of injury depends on the following except _____.

    A. body and surface features

    B. the manner of body impacts onto the surface

    C. the surface of high deformity

5. The proportion of _____ in the elderly population is twice of the average.

    A. falling   B. fractures   C. home-accident

ER-11-3
扫一扫 听一听

ER-11-4
扫一扫 知情节

Part B

Words in Focus

independence /ˌindiˈpendəns/	*n.*	独立；自主；自立
capability /ˌkeipəˈbiləti/	*n.*	能力；才能；才干
achievement /əˈtʃivmənt/	*n.*	成就，功绩
reinforcement /ˌriːinˈfɔːsmənt/	*n.*	增强，加强
caregiver /ˈkeəgivə(r)/	*n.*	照料者，护理者
limitation /ˈlimiˈteiʃn/	*n.*	限制，局限性
independently /ˌindiˈpɛndəntli/	*adv.*	独立地，自立地
supervision /ˌsjupɔˈviʒən/	*n.*	监督，管理
accomplishment /əˈkɑːmpliʃmənt/	*n.*	成就，完成，技艺

Useful Expressions

activities of daily living (ADLs)	日常生活活动
self-care activities	自我照顾活动
physical limitation	体力限度
contribute to	有助于

Text

Directions: In this section you will hear a short passage, at the end of the passage, one or more questions will be asked about what was said, decide which the best answer is.

ER-11-5
扫一扫 读一读

ER-11-6
扫一扫 看一看

笔记

ER-11-7
扫一扫 听一
听

ER-11-8
扫一扫 知情
节

Background:

    You are attending a CPD (Continuous Professional Development) training session given by a Clinical Nurse Specialist, Mr. David Hockings, on elderly management.

Comprehension of the text

1. What can the promoting independence in self-care of older adults do except?

    A. leave older adults with a sense of achievement

    B. provide older adults with the capability to maintain independence longer

    C. complete a task aided

2. Older adults that require assistance with ADLs are at a greater risk of _____.

    A. meeting with reinforcement from caregivers

    B. losing their independence with self-care tasks

    C. being conscious of actions and behaviors

3. It is important for caregivers to ensure that measures are put into place _____.

    A. to preserve and promote function

    B. to contribute to a decline in status in an older adult

    C. to become dependent on caregivers

4. Caregivers need to do followings except _____.

    A. perform self-care independently

    B. be conscious of actions and behaviors

    C. allow older patients to maintain as much independence as possible

5. Caregivers should encourage older adults in their efforts as _____.

    A. it can provide them with a sense of accomplishment

    B. it can't keep the ability to maintain independence longer

    C. they can't see the benefit in performing self-care independently

Part Ⅱ   Speaking

    This section is designed to test your speaking ability. After learning the following conversation A and B you will have the ability of speaking skill in medical and nursing working and try to do the following speaking tasks.

Conversation 1

Educating a Relative of a Patient with Alzheimer Disease

    Mr. Clausen, whose mother is a patient with Alzheimer's disease, is complaining of something wrong with his mother. Dr. Boland is listening and educating him about the symptoms and interventions for Alzheimer's disease.

ER-11-9
扫一扫 听一
听

ER-11-10
扫一扫 知情
节

笔记

Mr. Clausen:	I can't take this another day. Now I am being accused of stealing my mother's underwear.
Dr. Boland:	Oh, I understand. Your mother suffers from Alzheimer's disease. This must be a difficult time for you and your mother.
Mr. Clausen:	Could you tell me the details about Alzheimer's disease?
Dr. Boland:	Alzheimer's disease, also called dementia of the Alzheimer type, is a chronic disease. A patient who has Alzheimer's disease will struggle in it three to ten

years.

Mr. Clausen:	Ten years? Is it curable?
Dr. Boland:	No, it is incurable. Some famous persons, for example, Mrs. Margaret Hilda Thatcher and Ronald Wilson Reagan, died of this disease. I'm sorry to tell you this.
Mr. Clausen:	Oh, my poor mother! Would you like to tell me what I could do for her?
Dr. Boland:	In the early stage of Alzheimer's dementia the client complains of forgetfulness and has difficulty remembering appointments and addresses. Your mother has long-term memory loss and disorientation, which are the symptoms at the middle stage of Alzheimer's dementia. I'll prescribe some medication which will improve her memory.
Mr. Clausen:	Oh, I'll let her take medicine in time. What else could I do?
Dr. Boland:	Talk more about something happy in the past with her, and promote independence in her self-care as much as possible.
Mr. Clausen:	Promote independence? What do you mean?
Dr. Boland:	Independence in self-care can give her with a sense of achievement. So let her do self-care as much as possible. For example, when you tell her to brush her teeth, it may be necessary to give her step-by-step directions.
Mr. Clausen:	What can we do for her memory loss?
Dr. Boland:	Establish a routine schedule of activities for her. Call her name, tell her where she is, and state your name at each contact with her. It is particularly important in the care of a patient who has Alzheimer's disease to assess the patient's abilities on an on-going basis.
Mr. Clausen:	Yesterday my wife offered my mother breakfast, she said, "Oh no, honey, I have to wait until my husband gets here." But my father died six years ago. How can we manage?
Dr. Boland:	Tell her the truth and help her. For instance, "My dad died six years ago. Let me put milk on your cereal for you."
Mr. Clausen:	She always loses her way, even at home, she can't find the washroom. How to manage?
Dr. Boland:	When she goes for a walk, you or other persons must accompany her. She needs a bracelet or a necklace with your contact number in case of her wandering. On the wall hang up an electric clock with the date and o'clock alarm, and write signs on the door.
Mr. Clausen:	Where is the best place that my mother live in now?
Dr. Boland:	Of course, at home. It is very important to provide a predictable environment. Make home as safe and familiar as possible. Don't change the furnishings in the house, especially in your mother's room. But if you maybe think your mother is out of control and you can't take it anymore someday, we should explore alternative care settings for the patient.

(494 words)

ER-11-11
扫一扫 读一读

ER-11-12
扫一扫 看一看

Words in Focus

Alzheimer /'ælz'ɛmə/　　　　　　　　　　*n.*　　　阿尔茨海默

笔记

dementia /dɪˈmɛnʃə/	n.	痴呆
struggle /ˈstrʌɡəl/	vi.	奋斗，挣扎
incurable /ʌnˈkjuərəbl/	adj.	不能治愈的
forgetfulness /fəˈɡetfəlnɪs/	n.	健忘
on-going /ˈɔnɡˈouɪŋ/	adj.	继续存在；不间断的
bracelet /ˈbreɪslət/	n.	手镯
necklace /ˈnɛklɪs/	n.	项链
wandering /ˈwɒndərɪŋ/	n.	漫游；流浪；漂泊；精神错乱
predictable /prɪˈdɪktəbl/	adj.	可预知的；可预报的
furnishing /ˈfənɪʃɪŋ/	n.	家具，设备，陈设品，服饰品
alternative /ɔːlˈtɜːrnətɪv/	adj.	二者择一的

Useful Expressions

Alzheimer's disease	阿尔茨海默病
step-by-step direction	一步一步的指导
memory loss	记忆丧失
a routine schedule	日常生活时间表
care settings	护理机构

I. Free talk

Directions: Work in pairs and discuss the following questions after listening to the recording of Dialogue One.

1. Explain to your partner how to care for patients with Alzheimer's disease?

_____

_____

2. What are the problems of Mr. Clausen's mother?

_____

_____

II. Comprehension of the text

Directions: Complete the sentences according to the text.

1. Alzheimer's disease, also called dementia of the Alzheimer type, is _____ disease.

　　A. an acute　　　　　　B. a chronic　　　　　　C. an infectious

2. Independence in self-care can give patients with a sense of _____.

　　A. shame　　　　　　　B. achievement　　　　　C. failure

3. In the early stage of Alzheimer's dementia the client complains of _____.

　　A. long-term memory loss　B. forgetfulness　　　C. disorientation

4. Establish a _____ schedule of activities for patients with Alzheimer's disease.

　　A. changeable　　　　　B. uncertain　　　　　　C. routine

5. It is very important to provide a _____ environment.

　　A. stimulating　　　　　B. predictable　　　　　C. restricted

ER-11-13
扫一扫 答案
"晓"

Conversation 2

A Consultation for an Elderly Patient with Major Depression

Dr. Smith, a psychiatrist, Barbara, a nursing specialist, and Tina, a ward nurse are talking about Mr. Williams, an 85-year-old patient with major depression.

笔记

| Dr. Smith: | Let's start with Mr. Williams. He is an 85-year-old patient who lives alone with hypertension and diabetes. He is an optimistic person before his wife died three months ago. He was used to walking, fishing, dancing and drinking every day. He lost all interest on anything outside him. Two days ago, he committed suicide and was discovered by his next door neighbor. He is diagnosed with major depression. Barbara, what are your observations on him? |

ER-11-14
扫一扫 听一听

ER-11-15
扫一扫 知情节

Barbara:	Depression is commonly associated with severe, chronic medical disorders and a recent loss. He lost his wife and suffered from hypertension and diabetes. Mr. Williams has depression, inhibition of thought and hypobulia or abulia.
Dr. Smith:	What is your care plan?
Barbara:	Because he is newly admitted for treatment of a major depression, the most appropriate intervention is short, frequent interactions. Tina, have you visited Mr. Williams?
Tina:	Yes, but he told me, "I'm too depressed to talk to you. Leave me alone."
Barbara:	What did you say?
Tina:	I said to him, "I'll sit here with you for a moment." I visit him once half an hour and sit with him for five minutes a time.
Barbara:	OK, very well. That was the most therapeutic response by a nurse. Did he tell you anything?
Tina:	He told me he would not be a problem much longer.
Barbara:	Oh, he still wants to die!
Dr. Smith:	Make sure maintaining a safe milieu should be included because most of patients with depression will commit suicide with a precise suicidal plan. What are the next interventions?
Barbara:	We'll give him a one-to-one observation if we find he has a plan for suicide. Can you order some antidepressant for him, Mr. Smith?
Dr. Smith:	Yes, I'll write up some medication. But pay attention to the side effects of medication, such as bradycardia, orthostatic hypotension, and arrhythmia.
Barbara:	OK, Mr. Smith. Do you remember other nursing actions for patients with major depression, Tina?
Tina:	They are group involvement, exploring negative feelings and teaching problem solving.
Barbara:	Which nursing action would be most effective when encouraging a depressed patient to be less socially isolated?
Tina:	Group involvement, it is much better to ask a more stable patient to accompany the patient to activities.
Dr. Smith:	If Mr. Williams is being prepared for discharge, which nursing action would be most therapeutic initially?
Barbara:	We'll refer him to social services.
Tina:	Social services will order something, such as enrolling him in a day-care center or arranging for food delivery by a home-delivered meals program if necessary.

笔记

Dr. Smith:　　Thank you for giving information.

(433 words)

Words in Focus

ER-11-16
扫一扫 读一读

consultation /ˌkɒnsəlˈteɪʃn/	n.	会诊；请教，咨询
depression /dɪˈprɛʃən/	n.	抑郁（症）
optimistic /ˌɒptɪˈmɪstɪk/	adj.	乐观的
hypobulia /haipoʊˈbjuːliə/	n.	意志薄弱，意志消沉
abulia /əˈbjuːliə/	n.	意志缺失
interaction /ˌɪntɔˈækʃən/	n.	相互作用
milieu /miːˈljə/	n.	环境
antidepressant /ˌæntidiˈprɛsənt/	n.	抗抑郁药
bradycardia /brædiˈkɑːdiə/	n.	心动过缓
involvement /inˈvɑːlvmənt/	n.	牵连，参与；加入

ER-11-17
扫一扫 看一看

Useful Expressions

major depression	重度抑郁（症）
commit suicide	自杀
inhibition of thought	思维抑制
side effect	副作用
orthostatic hypotension	直立性低血压，体位性低血压
day-care center	日间护理中心

I. Free talk

Directions: *Work in pairs and discuss the following questions after learning to the Conversation Two.*

1. Explain to your partner how to care the patients with major depression?

_____

_____

2. What are the problems of Mr. Williams?

_____

_____

II. Comprehension of the text

Directions: *Complete the sentences according to the conversation.*

1. Mr. Williams committed _____ two days ago.

　　A. a treatment　　　　　　B. suicide　　　　　　C. a crime

2. _____ is commonly associated with severe, chronic medical disorders.

　　A. Hypertension　　　　　B. Depression　　　　　C. Diabetes

3. A(n) _____ observation is suitable for a depression patient with a plan for suicide.

　　A. immediate　　　　　　B. one-to-one　　　　　C. indirect

4. The side effects of antidepressant are bradycardia, _____, arrhythmia.

　　A. orthostatic hypotension

　　B. vascular hypotension

　　C. idiopathic hypotension

5. Which would be the most effective nursing action when encouraging a depressed patient to be less socially isolated?

ER-11-18
扫一扫 答案
"晓"

笔 记

A. Exploring negative feelings
B. Teaching problem solving
C. Group involvement

Part Ⅲ   Reading

Text A

The distinguishing marks associated with the elderly comprise both physical and mental characteristics. A basic mark of old age that affects both body and mind is "slowness of behavior".

Pre-reading

1. What is human aging?
2. How to prevent pulmonary complications in the elderly?
3. Why should older people be taught to walk steadily?

ER-11-19
扫一扫 听一听

ER-11-20
扫一扫 知情节

The Musculoskeletal System of the Elderly

Human aging is a gradually systemic degenerative process of every part in a human body, which includes the degeneration of the musculoskeletal system. Companying with the aging, there is a decrease or a decline in both muscles and bones.

After 30 years old, the size and number of muscle fibers decrease consistently, and their declines become more rapid after age 50. Muscle flexibility and elasticity degenerates simultaneously which can result in some dysfunction even diseases. For example, decreased elasticity in the chest muscles and cartilage between ribs makes the volume of lung expansion and the reserve capacity smaller. So the elderly may tire more quickly and get pneumonia more easily than younger. To avoid fatigue, their activities should be spread out and paced as much as possible. Some interventions, such as early treatment of colds and flu, good nutrition, adequate exercise, no smoking and deep breathing, can prevent pulmonary complications. It is important to know there are two changes in muscles about the elderly. Firstly, smaller muscles' declines imply the older people have less storage of glycogen, which means they have a slower reaction to emergency and risk. Secondly, the elderly especially women who have delivered children are made hard to control passing urine in their later years because of decreased muscle tone.

Between 18 and 30 years old, bones attain their maximum density, but after that time they begin to lose mass and become less dense or more porous, which is more rapidly in women than in men. Loss of bone density in the vertebral discs brings about the elderly to lose height and to have a tendency towards stooped posture. A spinal curvature known as kyphosis can occur. Changes in posture and gait result from changes in the long bones and spinal column, and make older people less stable and balanced when walking. Body sway increases with age and changes equilibrium and balance. In order to give them a better base or support and to compensate sway, older people should be taught to walk using a wide walk.

Osteoporosis is known as an extreme thinning and brittleness of bone. Some factors, such

笔记

as decreased oestrogen levels, smoking, alcohol, lack of exercise, calcium deficiency, early menopause, possible changes in protein metabolism and frequent use of steroids, contribute to it. Whether osteoporosis is considered to be a typical age-related change or an illness probably depends on the degree of osteoporosis. Osteoarthritis, also known as degenerative arthritis, is a non-inflammatory deterioration of joints, which begins with thinning and loss of cartilage, and progresses to more complete loss of cartilage and the formation of bone spurs. Beyond 60 years of age, about 25% of women and 15% of men have symptoms of osteoarthritis and by 75 years of age, as many as 85% may have evidence of the disease.

(467 words)

Words in Focus

musculoskeletal /ˌmʌskjəlouˈskelitəl/	*adj.*	肌（与）骨骼的
degenerative /diˈdʒɛnərətiv/	*adj.*	退步的，变质的，退化的
degeneration /diˌdʒenəˈreiʃn/	*n.*	变性，退化，变质
decline /diˈklain/	*n.*	减退期，衰退
consistently /kənˈsistəntli/	*adv.*	一贯地，始终如一地
flexibility /ˌflɛksiˈbiliti/	*n.*	屈曲性
elasticity /elæˈstisiti/	*n.*	弹性
degenerate /diˈdʒenəreit/	*vi./adj.*	退化 / 退化的
simultaneously /simlˈteiniəsli/	*adv.*	同时地
dysfunction /disˈfʌŋkʃən/	*n.*	机能不良，功能紊乱
cartilage /ˈkɑːtilidʒ/	*n.*	软骨
pulmonary /ˈpʌlmənri/	*adj.*	肺部的
glycogen /ˈglaikədʒən/	*n.*	糖原
density /ˈdɛnsiti/	*n.*	密度
porous /ˈpɔrəs/	*adj.*	多孔的
stooped /ˈstuːp/	*adj.*	弯腰的
curvature /ˈkɜːrvətʃə(r)/	*n.*	弯曲
kyphosis /kaiˈfousis/	*n.*	驼背
equilibrium /ˌikwəˈlibriəm/	*n.*	平衡，平静
compensate /ˈkɑːmpenseit/	*vi.*	偿还，补偿
sway /swe/	*n.*	摇摆，摇动
osteoporosis /ˌɑːstioupəˈrousis/	*n.*	骨质疏松症
brittleness /ˈbritlnəs/	*n.*	脆性，脆度；脆弱性
oestrogen /ˈɛstrədʒən/	*n.*	雌激素
menopause /ˌmɛnəˈpɔz/	*n.*	绝经期，更年期
osteoarthritis /ˌɑːstiouɑːrˈθraitis/	*n.*	骨关节炎
arthritis /ɑːrˈθraitis/	*n.*	关节炎
spur /spə/	*n.*	骨刺，骨距

Useful Expressions

musculoskeletal system	肌肉骨骼系统
muscle tone	肌肉张力
vertebral disc	椎间盘
a wide walk	宽步行走

笔记

non-inflammatory deterioration　　　　　　非炎性退化

spinal column　　　　　　　　　　　　　脊柱

Post-reading

I. Comprehension of the text

Ⅰ) **Choose the best answer to complete each sentence with the information from the text.**

1. After _____ years old the size and number of muscle fibers decreases consistently, and their declines become more rapid after age _____.

A. 50, 30　　　　　　　　B. 30, 30　　　　　　　　C. 30, 50

2. Decreased elasticity in the chest muscles and cartilage between ribs makes the volume of lung _____ and the reserve capacity _____.

A. expansion, large　　　B. contraction, smaller　　C. expansion, smaller

3. Early treatment of colds and flu, good nutrition, adequate exercise, no smoking and deep breathing, can prevent pulmonary complications.

A. yes　　　　　　　　　B. no　　　　　　　　　　C. not mentioned

4. After _____ bones begin to lose mass and become less dense or more porous.

A. 30 years old　　　　　B. 40 years old　　　　　C. 50 years old

5. Beyond 60 years of age, about _____ of women and _____ of men have symptoms of osteoarthritis.

A. 25%, 20%　　　　　　B. 25%, 15%　　　　　　C. 35%, 15%

Ⅱ) **Read the following statements and then decide whether each of them is true or false based on the information from the text. Write T for true and F for false in the space provided.**

_____ 1. Human aging is a gradually systemic degenerative process of every part in a human body.

_____ 2. The size and number of muscle fibers decreases consistently, and their declines become more rapid after age 50.

_____ 3. In order to give them a better base or support and to compensate sway, older people shouldn't be taught to walk using a wide walk.

_____ 4. Whether osteoporosis is considered to be a typical age-related change or an illness probably depends on the degree of osteoarthritis.

II. Vocabulary activities

Find a word or phrase from the box below to complete each sentence. There are more words and phrases than you need to fill in all the sentences. Change word forms where necessary.

osteoarthritis	flexibility	degeneration	pneumonia	glycogen
curvature	osteoporosis	elasticity	kyphosis	menopause
disfunction	musculoskeletal system			

1. Human aging includes the _____ of the _____.
2. Muscle _____ and _____ degenerates simultaneously.
3. The elderly may get _____ more easily than younger.
4. The older people have less storage of _____.
5. A spinal _____ known as _____ can occur in the elderly.
6. _____ is known as an extreme thinning and brittleness of bone.
7. _____ is a non-inflammatory deterioration of joints.

笔记

III. Supplementary

Text B

> Hip replacement is currently the most common orthopaedic operation. The aims of the procedure are pain relief and improvement in hip function.
>
> ### Pre-reading
> 1. What is hip replacement?
> 2. What are do's and don'ts after hip replacement?

Guidelines of Daily Living about Hip Replacement

Hip replacement is a surgical procedure in which the hip joint is replaced by a prosthetic implant. Hip replacement surgery can be performed as a total replacement or a hemi replacement. Such joint replacement orthopaedic surgery is generally conducted to relieve arthritis pain or in some hip fractures.

The day of hip replacement surgery is mostly a day to recover from procedure, but it is not just about rest. Depending on the time of day of surgery, the patient may be asked to sit in a chair or on the side of the bed. Patients will begin simple activities including ankle pumps, leg lifts, and heel slides. It is important for patients to take sufficient pain medication and to allow them to participate in their rehabilitation exercises.

During hospitalization, patients will meet with physical and occupational therapists. The physiotherapist will work on mobility, strengthening and walking. The occupational therapist will work on preparing for tasks such as washing, dressing, and other daily activities. Factors that will affect the rate of progression include patients' strength before surgery, body weight, and ability to manage painful symptoms. The type and extent of surgery can also affect their ability to participate in physical therapy.

After hip replacement surgery, some precautions, known as "hip precautions", are necessary to protect the newly implanted hip. Hip precautions prevent the patient from placing their hip in a position where the ball could potentially come out of the socket — a problem called a hip dislocation.

Patients are usually discharged 3 to 5 days after hip replacement surgery. Most patients take their first steps after surgery with the aid of a walker. Patients with good balance and a strong upper body may opt to use crutches. Transitioning to a cane depends on two factors. First one is restrictions from surgeon — not all surgeons allow full weight to be placed on the leg in the early weeks after surgery. Second is patients' ability to regain strength. Many patients have to navigate stairs in order to enter or get through their homes. Therefore, the therapist will work with his patient to get up and down steps using crutches or a walker.

Return to driving depends on a number of factors including the side of operation and the type of vehicle the patients have (standard or automatic). Patients need to be able to safely and quickly operate the gas and brake pedals. Under no circumstances should patients drive when taking narcotic pain medications. Patients can resume sexual activity once comfortable. It is important that patients maintain their usual hip precautions to avoid dangerous positions. Return to work depends on the activity that patients have to do at their job. Patients who work in a seated position, with limited walking, can plan on returning within about 4 weeks from the time of surgery. Patients who are more active at work may need more time until they can return to full duties.

(489 words)

Words in Focus

replacement /rɪˈpleɪsmənt/	*n.*	置换
prosthetic /prɒsˈθɛtɪk/	*adj.*	假体的
orthopaedic /ˌɔːθəʊˈpiːdɪk/	*adj.*	整形外科的
rehabilitation /ˌriːhəˌbɪlɪˈteɪʃən/	*n.*	复原，恢复，康复
physiotherapist /ˌfɪziəʊˈθerəpɪst/	*n.*	理疗师
mobility /məʊˈbɪləti/	*n.*	可动性，移动性
socket /ˈsɑːkɪt/	*n.*	窝，穴，孔
dislocation /ˌdɪsləˈkeɪʃən/	*n.*	脱位
walker /ˈwɔːkə/	*n.*	助步架，步行器
transition /trænˈzɪʃən/	*n.*	转换，过渡，变迁
navigate /ˈnævɪˈgeɪt/	*vt.*	横渡，跨越
crutch /krʌtʃ/	*n.*	拐杖，支器
standard /ˈstændəd/	*n./adj.*	标准规格 / 标准的
automatic /ˌɔːtəˈmætɪk/	*adj.*	自动的
narcotic /nɑːˈkɒtɪk/	*n./adj.*	麻醉药 / 麻醉的

ER-11-27
扫一扫 读一读

ER-11-28
扫一扫 看一看

Useful Expressions

hip replacement	髋关节置换
prosthetic implant	假体性植入物
occupational therapist	职业治疗师

Post-reading

I. Comprehension of the text

Ⅰ) **Choose the best answer to complete each sentence with the information from the text.**

1. Patients are usually discharged _____ days after hip replacement surgery.

    A. 2 to 3　　　　　　B. 3 to 5　　　　　　C. 5 to 7

2. A problem called a _____ refers that the ball comes out of the socket.

    A. hip replacement　　　B. hip dislocation　　　C. prosthetic implant

3. Patients with good balance and a strong upper body may opt to use _____.

    A. cane　　　　　　　B. walker　　　　　　C. crutches

4. Patients who work in a seated position, with limited walking, can plan on returning within about _____ weeks from the time of surgery.

    A. 5　　　　　　　　B. 4　　　　　　　　C. 3

5. Patients may not be able to return to activities such as roofing after hip replacement.

    A. Right　　　　　　B. Wrong　　　　　　C. Not mentioned

Ⅱ) **Read the following statements and then decide whether each of them is true or false based on the information from the text. Write T for true and F for false in the space provided.**

_____ 1. Hip replacement surgery can be performed as a half replacement or a hemi replacement.

_____ 2. It is important for patients to take sufficient pain medication to allow them to

笔记

169

participate in their rehabilitation exercises.

_____ 3. The physiotherapist will work on mobility, strengthening, and washing.

_____ 4. Under no circumstances should patients drive when taking narcotic pain medications.

II. Vocabulary activities

Find a word or phrase from the box below to complete each sentence. There are more words and phrases than you need to fill in all the sentences. Change word forms where necessary.

hip fracture	dislocation	mobility	hospitalization	physical
occupational	precautions	arthritis	transitioning	prosthetic implant
hip replacement		orthopaedic surgery		

1. _____ is a surgical procedure in which the hip joint is replaced by a _____.
2. Such joint replacement _____ is generally conducted to relieve _____ pain or in some _____.
3. During _____, patients will meet with _____ and _____ therapists.
4. After hip replacement surgery, some _____ are necessary to protect the newly implanted hip.
5. _____ to a cane depends on two factors.

III. Supplementary

Part IV Writing

Writing a Package Insert

Instructions:

A **package insert** (formally **prescribing information** in the United States; in Europe, **Patient information leaflet** for human medicines or **package leaflet** for veterinary medicines) is a document provided along with a prescription or over-the-counter medication to provide additional information about that drug.

Package inserts follow a standard format for every medication and include the same types of information. The first thing listed is usually **the brand name** and **generic name** of the product. The other sections are as follows:

Clinical pharmacology tells how the medicine works in the body, how it is absorbed and eliminated, and what its effects are likely to be at various concentrations. It may also contain results of various clinical trials (studies) and/or explanations of the medication's effect on various populations (e.g. children, women, etc.).

Indications and usage uses (indications) for which the drug has been FDA-approved (e.g. migraines, seizures, high blood pressure). Physicians legally can and often do prescribe medicines for purposes not listed in this section (so-called "off-label uses").

Contraindications lists situations in which the medication should not be used, for example in patients with other medical conditions such as kidney problems or allergies.

Warnings covers possible serious side effects that may occur.

Precautions explains how to use the medication safely including physical impairments and drug interactions; for example "Do not drink alcohol while taking this medication".

ER-11-29
扫一扫 答案
"晓"

ER-11-30
扫一扫 练一
练

笔记

Adverse reactions lists all side effects observed in all studies of the drug (as opposed to just the dangerous side effects which are separately listed in "Warnings" section).

Drug abuse and dependence provides information regarding whether prolonged use of the medication can cause physical dependence (only included if applicable).

Overdosage gives the results of an overdose and provides recommended action in such cases.

Dosage and administration - gives recommended dosage(s); may list more than one for different conditions or different patients (e.g., lower dosages for children)

How supplied explains in detail the physical characteristics of the medication including color, shape, markings, etc., and storage information (e.g., "Do not store above 95℃")

Sentence Patterns:

1. Benemid is recommended for the treatment of gout, and to increase and prolong the plasma concentration of penicillins during anti-infective therapy.
   丙磺舒被推荐用于治疗痛风及在抗感染治疗时增加并延长青霉素类的血浆浓度。

2. Adriamycin is frequently used in combination chemotherapy regiments with other cytotoxic drugs.
   阿霉素常与其他细胞毒药物合用于化疗方案。

3. Amikacin is useful in the treatment of infections from Gram-negative sensitive species; It may also be useful to treat infections caused by sensitive staphylococci.
   阿米卡星可用于治疗革兰阳性敏感菌（其中包括假单孢菌）引起的感染，也可用于治疗敏感葡萄球菌引起的感染。

4. Children under 5 years of age should not be treated with Antistine.
   5岁以下儿童禁用（敌胺）安他啉。

5. This product is contraindicated in those patients who have shown hypersensitivity to it.
   对本品过敏的病人禁用。

6. Ursosan should not be given to patients suffering from bile duct obstruction.
   胆管阻塞病人禁用熊去氧胆酸。

7. It is advisable to avoid the use of Aramine with cyclo-propane, unless clinical circumstances demand such use.
   如果不是临床需要，建议阿拉明不要与环丙烷合用。

8. Do not take this medication if you are currently taking MAOI inhibitors.
   如果你当前正在服用单氧化酶抑制剂不要服用此药。

9. The tablets (or the syrup) are to be taken during or after a meal with a little liquid.
   片剂（或糖浆）应于食间或饭后用少量液体送服。

10. The initial dosage recommended is ½ tablet of Madopa three times daily.
    美多巴初始剂量推荐为每日3次，每次半片。

11. The recommended starting dose is 20 mg given as a single daily dose.
    推荐的首剂量为每日20mg，一次服用。

12. For adults given intramuscular injection of 400 to 600 mg per day in 2 to 3 divided doses.
    成年人肌内注射，每日400～600mg，分2～3次注射。

13. Packs (Madopa): cross-scored tablets each containing 200mg levodopa and 50mg benserazide.
    包装（美多巴刻痕片）每片含200mg左旋多巴和50mg苄丝肼。

14. Trade packs containing 50 and 100 sugar coated tablets.

商品包装：包括 50 及 100 片糖衣片。

15. Packs Standard packs of 20 dregees; Hospital packs of 100, 500 and 1000dregees.

   包装标准：包装为 20 粒糖衣丸，医院用包装为 100，500 及 1000 粒糖衣丸。

16. Also available in Hospital Unit-Dose blister package of 100.

   也提供医院用的单位剂量的铝塑包装，（每包）100 片装。

17. Do not store the suppositories over 25℃.

   本栓剂不得存于 25℃ 以上的温度。

18. Validity and storage: the solution will keep for five years if stored at a temperature below 20℃.

   有效期及贮存方法：溶液放置于 20℃ 以下可保存 5 年。

19. The solution should be prepared immediately prior to use, but can be stored at 4℃ up to one week.

   药液应在配制后立即使用，但在 4℃ 下可贮存一周。

Examples:

Approval date: Dec.26,2006

Insert of Trimetazidine Dihydrochloride Tablets

Carefully read insert and conform to the physician's prescription.

/ Drug names /

Generic name: Trimetazidine dihydrochloride tablets

Trade name: VASOREL®

English name: Trimetazidine Dihydrochloride Tablets (VASOREL®)

Chinese Pinyin: Yansuan Qumeitaqin Pian

/ Ingredients /

Chemical name: Trimetazidine dihydrochloride, 1-(2,3,4-trimethoxybenzyl) piperazine dihydrochloride

Structural formula:

Molecular formula: C14H22N2O3•2HCl

Molecular weight: 339.3

/ Description / Film-coated tablet with white core

/ Indications /

Prophylactic treatment of episodes of angina pectoris. Adjuvant symptomatic treatment of vertigo and tinnitus.

Rare cases of gastrointestinal disorders (nausea and vomiting).

Because of the presence of sunset yellow FCF S (E110) and cochineal red A (E124), risk of allergic reactions.

/ Contraindications /

This drug should never be used in case of hypersensitivity to any one of the product's constituents. This drug is generally not recommended during breastfeeding (Cf. Pregnancy and lactation).

/ Precautions /

This drug is not a curative treatment for angina attacks, nor is it indicated as initial treatment for unstable angina, or myocardial infarction. It should not be used in the pre-hospital phase nor during the first days of hospitalization; In the event of an angina attack, the coronaropathy should be reevaluated and an adaptation of the treatment considered (drug treatment and possibly revascularisation).

/ Pregnancy and lactation /

Pregnancy: Studies in animals have not demonstrated a teratogenic effect ; however, in the absence of clinical data, the risk of malformation cannot be excluded. Therefore, for safety reasons, it is preferable to avoid prescription during pregnancy.

Breast feeding: In the absence of data on excretion in breast milk, breastfeeding is not recommended during treatment.

/ Use in Children /

Safety and effectiveness in pediatric patients have not been established.

/ Use in Elderly /

See information in other items or follow physician's instructions.

/ Interactions of drugs /

In order to avoid possible interactions between various medicines, you must always tell your doctor or pharmacist about any other treatment you are receiving.

/ Over dosage /

It is important that you respect the doses prescribed by your doctor. If you think that the effects of Vasorel is too strong or too weak, talk to your doctor.

If you suspect that you have taken more than the amount of Vasorel prescribed by your doctor, contact your doctor immediately.

Do not take a double dose to make up for a forgotten dose, just carry on with the next dose at the usual time.

/ Pharmacology /

Other cardiovascular antianginal drug.

By preserving energy metabolism in cells exposed to hypoxia or ischaemia, trimetazidine prevents a decrease in intracellular ATP levels, thereby ensuring the proper functioning of ionic pumps and transmembrane sodium-potassium flow whilst maintaining cellular homeostasis.

In animals:

Trimetazidine:

- helps maintain energy metabolism in the heart and neurosensory organs during episodes of is chaemia and hypoxia.

- reduces intracellular acidosis and alterations in transmembrane ion flow caused by ischaemia.

- decreases the migration and infiltration of polynuclear neutrophils in ischaemic and reperfused cardiac tissue.

It also reduces the size of experimental infarctions.

- exerts this action in the absence of any direct haemodynamic effect.

In man:

Controlled studies in angina patients have shown that trimetazidine :

- increases coronary flow reserve, thereby delaying the onset of exercise-induced is chaemia, starting from the 15th day of treatment.

- limits rapid swings in blood pressure without any significant variations in heart rate.

- significantly decreases the frequency of angina attacks.

- leads to a significant decrease in the use of trinitroglycerin.

/ **Pharmacokinetics** /

- After oral administration, absorption of trimetazidine is rapid and the plasma peak is reached in less than 2 hours.

- After a single oral dose of 20mg of trimetazidine, the peak plasma concentration is about 55 ng/ml.

- During repeated administration, the steady state is reached after 24 to 36 hours and remains very stable throughout treatment.

- The apparent distribution volume is 4.8 L/kg which suggests good tissue diffusion. Protein binding is low ; in vitro measurements give a value of 16%.

- Trimetazidine is eliminated primarily in the urine, mainly in the unchanged form.

- The elimination half-life is approximately 6 hours.

/ **Storage** /　　below 30℃

/ **Package** /　　Alu-Alu blister; 15, 30, 60 tablets/box

/ **Shelf life** /　　36 months

/ **Specification No.** /　　YBH13562005

/ **Approval No.** /　　国药准字 H20055465

/ **Manufacturer** /

Servier（Tianjin）Pharmaceutical Company Limited

12, 10 th Avenue, Economic Technological & Development Area,Tianjin

Zip code:300457

Tel: (8622) 66299458

Fax: (8622) 66299456

Representative Office:

Servier International Beijing Office

Room B801, Han Wei Plaza,

No. 7 Guanghua Road,

Chaoyang District, Beijing, P.R.C.

Zip code:100004

Tel: (8610) 65610341

Fax: (8610) 65610348

Web-site:www.servier.com.cn

Practice:

药品名称：

通用名称：氢溴酸加兰他敏片

英文名称：Galanthamine Hydrobromide Tablets

商品名称：奇尔能

笔记

适应证：

本品适用于良性记忆障碍，提高病人指向记忆、联想学习、及人像回忆等能力。对痴呆患者和脑器质性病变引起的记忆障碍亦有改善作用。

用法用量：

口服，一次 5mg，一日 4 次；三天后改为一次 10mg，一日 4 次或遵医嘱。

不良反应：

神经系统：常见有疲劳、头晕眼花、头痛、发抖、失眠、梦幻。罕见有张力亢进、感觉异常、失语症和运动机能亢进等。

胃肠系统：腹涨、反胃、呕吐、腹痛、腹泻、厌食及体重减轻、消化不良等较常见。

禁忌：

对本品中任一成份过敏者禁用。加兰他敏为胆碱脂酶抑制剂，在麻醉的情况下禁止使用。心绞痛及心动过缓者禁用。严重哮喘或肺功能障碍的病人禁用。重度肝脏损害者禁用。重度肾脏损害者禁用。机械性肠梗。

注意事项：

有消化溃疡病史、或同时使用非甾体抗炎药的病人慎用。中度肝脏损害的病人慎用本品，必要时应适当减量。中度肾脏损害的病人慎用本品，必要时应减量使用。本品可能引起头晕、嗜睡，会影响驾驶及操作机械的能力。

FDA 妊娠药物分级：

尚未进行孕妇研究，但在动物繁殖性研究中，未见到对胎儿的影响，并且孕妇使用该药品的治疗获益可能胜于其潜在危害。或者，该药品尚未进行动物试验，也没有对孕妇进行充分严格的对照研究。

药物相互作用：

本品具有潜在的削弱抗胆碱功能药物治疗效果的作用。与类胆碱作用物以及其他胆碱脂酶抑制剂合用具有协同作用。本品与甲氰咪胍、酮康唑合用，可提高本品的生物利用度。与红霉素合用，可减低本品的疗效。

毒理研究：

加兰他敏是一个明确的具有选择性、竞争性及可逆性的乙酰胆碱脂酶抑制剂。另外还可提高体内乙酰胆碱对烟碱能受体的作用，其机制可能在于对烟碱型胆碱能受体进行变构调节。

生产企业：

丽珠集团丽珠制药厂

笔记

ER-11-31
扫一扫 答案
"晓"

Part V   Enriching your word power

1. presby(o)-; gerat(o)-; geront(o)-　　　　　　老年, 老人
   presbycusis /ˈprezbiˈkjuːsis/　　　　　　　　老年性耳聋
   presbyopia /ˌprezbiˈəupiə/　　　　　　　　　老花眼, 远视眼
   geratology /dʒerəˈtɒlədʒi/　　　　　　　　　老年医学, 老年病学
   geriatrist /ˌdʒeriˈætrist/　　　　　　　　　　老年病学者
   gerontology /ˌdʒerənˈtɒlədʒi/　　　　　　　老人医学
2. ocul(o)-; ophthalm(o)-; opt(o)-　　　　　　　眼
   oculist /ˈɒkjəlist/　　　　　　　　　　　　　眼科医生
   ophthalmology /ˌɒfθælˈmɒlədʒi/　　　　　　眼科学
   ophthalmocopia /ˌɒfθælməuˈkəupiə/　　　　　眼疲劳
   optometrist /ɒpˈtɒmitrist/　　　　　　　　　验光师, 视力测定者
3. retin(o)-　　　　　　　　　　　　　　　　　视网膜
   retinodialysis /retiˈnəudjəlisis/　　　　　　　视网膜剥离
   retinopathy /retiˈnɒpəθi/　　　　　　　　　　视网膜病
4. conjunctive(o)-　　　　　　　　　　　　　　结膜
   conjunctivitis /kənˌdʒʌŋktiˈvaitis/　　　　　结膜炎
   conjunctivoma /kəndˈʒʌŋktivəumə/　　　　　结膜瘤
5. corne(o)-　　　　　　　　　　　　　　　　　角膜
   cornea /ˈkɔːniə/　　　　　　　　　　　　　　角膜
   corneitis /ˌkɔːniˈaitis/　　　　　　　　　　　角膜炎
6. lacrim(o)-; dacry(o)-　　　　　　　　　　　　泪
   lacrimation /ˌlækriˈmeiʃən/　　　　　　　　　流泪
   dacrycystitis /ˌdækrikisˈtaitis/ 同 dacryocystitis　泪囊炎
7. aur(i)-; ot(o)-　　　　　　　　　　　　　　　耳
   auristilla /ɔːˈristilə/ (pl.auristillae)　　　　　滴耳剂
   otorrhea /əutəˈriːə/　　　　　　　　　　　　耳液溢出, 耳漏
8. scler(o)-　　　　　　　　　　　　　　　　　巩膜, 硬化
   scleroderma /ˌskliərəˈdɜːmə/　　　　　　　　硬皮病
   sclerotitis /skliərəuˈtaitis/　　　　　　　　　巩膜炎
9. acous(o)-; audi(o)-　　　　　　　　　　　　听觉, 听
   acousma /əˈkuːsmə/　　　　　　　　　　　　幻听

笔记

audiology /ˌɔːdiˈɒlədʒi/　　　　　　　听力学
10. gerontology /ˌdʒerənˈtɒlədʒi/　　　老年病学
　　presbycusis /ˌprezbiˈkjuːsis/　　　老年性耳聋
　　glaucoma /ɡlɔːˈkəumə/　　　　　　青光眼
　　hyperopia /ˌhaipəˈrəupiə/　　　　远视
　　Alzheimer's dementia　　　　　　阿尔茨海默病（老年痴呆）
　　Parkinson disease /ˈpɑːkinsən/　　帕金森病
　　memory loss　　　　　　　　　　失忆，健忘
　　recent memory loss　　　　　　　近期记忆丧失
　　remote memory loss　　　　　　　远期记忆丧失

Part Ⅵ　Exercise

Directions: In this section, only one of the following options is correct, please choose.

（罗晓冰　吕小君）

ER-11-32
扫一扫 看一
看

笔记

Unit 12
Surgery Department

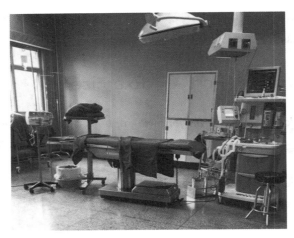

Fig. 12-1   surgery department

An ounce of prevention is worth a pound of cure.

一分预防胜过十分治疗。

Learning Objectives

Skill focus

1. Master aseptic procedures.
2. Master how to give instructions to a patient before and after a surgery of appendicitis and fracture.
3. Know the nursing care required to safely care for patients undergoing surgery.
4. Understand the overview on perioperative and immobilization.

Language focus

1. Aseptic dressing technique.
2. Have ability of creating and guessing a new word using roots and prefix or suffix.

Part I   Listening

This section is designed to test your ability to understand spoken English in nursing or medical contexts. You will hear a selection of recorded materials and you must answer the questions that accompany them. There are TWO parts in this section, Part A and Part B.

Part A

Words in Focus

aseptic /əˈsɛptɪk, e-/   adj.   <术>无菌的；经消毒的

microbial /maɪˈkroʊbiəl/	*adj.*	微生物的，由细菌引起的
contamination /kənˌtæmɪˈneɪʃən/	*n.*	污染
trolley /ˈtrɑːli/	*n.*	治疗车
integrate /ˈɪntɪˌɡreɪt/	*adj.*	完整的
sterilize /ˈstɛrəlaɪz/	*vt.*	消毒；使无菌
sterile /ˈstɛraɪl/	*adj.*	无菌的
clip /klɪp/	*v.*	用别针别在某物上，用夹子夹在某物上

ER-12-1
扫一扫 读一读

Useful Expressions

post-operative	术后的
aseptic procedures	无菌操作
aseptic dressing technique	无菌更换敷料技术
sterile packaging	无菌包
nursing notes	护理记录

ER-12-2
扫一扫 看一看

Text

Directions: *In this section you will hear a short passage, at the end of the passage, one or more questions will be asked about what was said, decide which the best answer is.*

Background:

   Mrs. Cameron, a 64-year-old lady, was admitted to the hospital a week ago. She has had an operation for back pain. She requires a post-operative care. In order to help her wound heal successfully, Julia, the in charge nurse, will show the nurse students some aseptic procedures through aseptic dressing technique.

ER-12-3
扫一扫 听一听

Comprehension of the text

1. Asepsis can be defined as "the prevention of microbial contamination of the following except _____".

   A. blood pressure   B. living tissue   C. sterile materials

2. Which need not be checked before using the sterile package?

   A. secure seals   B. the integrity   C. weight

3. Where did Jane put the necessary sterile packaging?

   A. in the laboratory   B. in the blood station   C. in the trolley

4. Does the sterile packaging need to be within expiry date?

   A. yes   B. no   C. not mentioned

5. Which of the following can check Mrs. Cameron's identification?

   A. gadget   B. ID bracelet   C. chart

ER-12-4
扫一扫 知情节

Part B

Words in Focus

gallipot /ˈɡæliˌpɒt/	*n.*	陶罐，药罐
discoloration /dɪsˌkʌləˈreɪʃən/	*n.*	变色，褪色
particle /ˈpɑːrtɪkl/	*n.*	微粒，颗粒
cloudiness /ˈklaʊdɪnɪs/	*n.*	混沌
saline /ˈseɪlaɪn/	*n.*	盐水；生理盐水

ER-12-5
扫一扫 读一读

ER-12-6
扫一扫 看一看

笔记

Useful Expressions

sterile field	无菌区
normal saline	生理盐水
expiry date	有效期
treatment room	治疗室

Text

Directions: *In this section you will hear a short passage, at the end of the passage, one or more questions will be asked about what was said, decide which the best answer is.*

Background:

　　All the students follow the head nurse to the treatment room.

Comprehension of the text

1. What should the nurse do before changing the patient's wound dressing?
   A. wash hands and wear the aprons
   B. identify the patient and lay out a sterile field
   C. All of the above
2. Which part of the pack should be opened first?
   A. The upper corner　　　B. The left corner　　　C. The inner corner
3. What did the head nurse put into the gallipot?
   A. enema　　　　　　　B. sedative　　　　　　C. saline
4. Which of the following is not the requirement for checking the normal saline bottle?
   A. no cracks　　　　　　B. no liquid　　　　　　C. no discoloration
5. The inside of which glove can't be touched when putting it up?
   A. the right one　　　　　B. the left one　　　　　C. both the right and left one

Part II　Speaking

　　This section is designed to test your speaking ability. After learning the following conversations A and B you will get some sense of what to say and what to hear in a hospital and try to do the following speaking tasks.

Conversation 1

Preoperative Nursing Care of Appendicitis

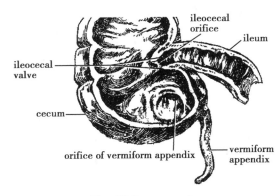

Fig. 12-2　appendix

ER-12-7
扫一扫 听一听

ER-12-8
扫一扫 知情节

ER-12-9
扫一扫 听一听

ER-12-10
扫一扫 知情节

笔记

180

One day, Mrs. Smith, the owner of a grocery shop, has a bad pain in her belly. She comes to the hospital and the registered nurse sends her to the emergency room immediately. Anne, the nurse of the emergency room asks her some questions for the case record. After taking her temperature the nurse gives her an examination of the belly and thinks that Mrs. Smith has got appendicitis. She reports to the doctor on duty and after having some tests the doctor decides to operate on Mrs. Smith at 10 o'clock. The doctor asks Anne to give Mrs. Smith an injection to release the pain first.

Nurse:	Good morning, Mrs. Smith. I heard in report that you will be having surgery at 10 o'clock.
Mrs. Smith:	Yes, I am a little nervous about it.
Nurse:	That is very normal. I'll give you an injection to relieve the pain first.
Mrs. Smith:	Thank you.
Nurse:	Now let me explain something about the surgery.
Mrs. Smith:	OK.
Nurse:	Now you will be NPO, which means you cannot eat or drink anything. It is important to keep your stomach empty before having general anesthesia.
Mrs. Smith:	Good. I will do that.
Nurse:	You will need to take off all your jewelry, watch, glasses and makeup. Before you leave for surgery, you will get some medicine to help you relax. And you will have an intravenous drip.
Mrs. Smith:	Well, I see. When will I be back to my room?
Nurse:	You should stay in the Recovery Room after the surgery until you are awake and alert. Then you can be back.
Mrs. Smith:	When will I have something to eat?
Nurse:	You will also be NPO until a day or two after surgery. When your bowels start working again, you will begin on a clear, then full liquid diet and progress to a regular diet.
Mrs. Smith:	That means I will eat nothing for almost two days?
Nurse:	Don't worry. You will have the intravenous fluid until you are eating. Also, after surgery we will be getting you up and out of bed very quickly and hourly during the day we will be encouraging you to cough and breathe deeply. These are important to help prevent any complications.
Mrs. Smith:	Won't it hurt to get out of bed and cough?
Nurse:	Yes, but you will have a pain medicine ordered. You need to ask for it. Any questions?
Mrs. Smith:	No, thanks a lot.
Nurse:	The doctor and anesthetist are ready now. Do you feel relaxed now?
Mrs. Smith:	I'm still a little afraid, but I feel better now.

(332 words)

Words in Focus

case /keis/	*n.*	病案，病例
appendicitis /əˌpɛndiˈsaitis/	*n.*	阑尾炎
anesthetist /əˈnɛsθətist/	*n.*	麻醉师
NPO（拉丁语）nil per os	*n.*	禁饮食
anesthesia /ˌænisˈθiːʒiə/	*n.*	麻醉

ER-12-11
扫一扫 读一读

ER-12-12
扫一扫 看一看

Useful Expressions

case record	病历，对患者病情、诊疗过程的记录
general anesthesia	全身麻醉
an intravenous drip	静脉滴注
the recovery room	手术后的特别病房，恢复室

I. Free talk

Directions: *Discuss with your teacher and your classmates what a patient who just underwent an operation for appendicitis should do and be careful about.*

_____

_____

II. Comprehension of Conversation 1

Directions: *Complete the sentences according to the conversation.*

1. What does NPO mean?

   A. no food　　　　　　B. no drink　　　　　　C. neither food nor drink

2. Did Mrs. Smith have to remove her makeup before surgery?

   A. yes　　　　　　　　B. no　　　　　　　　　C. not mentioned

3. Why did the nurse encourage Mrs. Smith to cough and breathe deeply?

   A. to help relieve constipation

   B. to prevent complications

   C. to relieve the pain

4. Until what time will Mrs. Smith have the intravenous fluid?

   A. She is awake.

   B. She is having general anesthesia.

   C. She is eating.

5. What if Mrs. Smith hurt to get out of bed and cough?

   A. have an injection　　B. have a pain medicine　　C. stay in bed all the time

ER-12-13
扫一扫 答案"晓"

Conversation 2

Elbow Fracture

   A patient fell on the ground and had an elbow fracture.

Doctor:　Hello! What is troubling you?

Patient:　I lost consciousness and fell on the ground. When I woke up, I felt a sharp pain in my right elbow. My elbow is badly swollen.

Doctor:　When did it happen?

Patient:　Three hours ago.

Doctor:　Is there any radiation of the pain to the shoulder?

Patient:　No. Er... I took a painkiller one hour ago.

Doctor:　Please roll up your sleeves. Point to the spot where you feel the most pain.

ER-12-14
扫一扫 听一听

ER-12-15
扫一扫 知情节

笔记

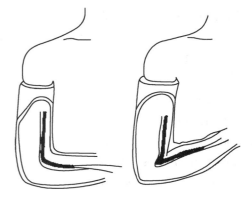

Fig. 12-3　elbow fracture

Patient: It's here, doctor. It has been stiff and looks black and blue. At times it feels numb.

Doctor: I'm afraid your right elbow joint is broken, we'd better X-ray it, just to be sure.

Patient: OK.

The nurse took the patient to the X-ray department.

Doctor: The X-ray shows a fracture of your elbow.

Patient: Doctor, will it heal properly?

Doctor: Cheer up. I think things will come all right.

Patient: Do I need an operation?

Doctor: Yeah, I think you'd better be hospitalized. We'll give you a "U" type plaster cast on your elbow.

Patient: OK.

Doctor: Keep your elbow higher than your heart for 24 to 72 hours.

Patient: Oh, I see.

Doctor: By the way, the cast should not be wet.

Patient: How long will I have to have the cast?

Doctor: About two months. And you'd better rest in bed after discharge. If you feel worse, Please come back to the hospital right away.

Patient: Thanks a lot.

(253 words)

Words in Focus

consciousness /ˈkɑːnʃəsnis/	*n.*	知觉；感觉
radiation /ˌreidiˈeiʃən/	*n.*	放射，辐射
painkiller /ˈpeinˌkilə/	*n.*	止痛药
stiff /stif/	*adj.*	僵硬的
heal /hiːl/	*v.*	（使）康复，复原

Useful Expressions

roll up	卷起
plaster cast	石膏模型；石膏绷带

I. Free talk

Directions: *If you are a nurse to help a patient take an X-ray, what are your considerations?*

_____

_____

II. Comprehension of the text

Directions: *Work in pairs and discuss the following questions after learning Conversation Two.*

1. Why does the patient need to have an X-ray?

_____

_____

2. What should be done on the patient's elbow to treat his fracture?

_____

_____

3. What should the patient do after discharge?

_____

_____

ER-12-16
扫一扫 读一
读

ER-12-17
扫一扫 看一
看

ER-12-18
扫一扫 答案
"晓"

笔 记

Part Ⅲ　Reading

Text A

> Perioperative nursing is a specialized nursing area wherein a registered nurse works as a team member of other surgical health care professionals. It describes the wide variety of nursing functions associated with the patient's surgical management.
>
> **Pre-reading**
> 1. What is the most important part of the peri-operative experience?
> 2. What is the goal of postoperative care?

Peri-operative Nursing

Peri-operative nursing is focused on care for patients undergoing any type of surgery. Peri-operative nursing is divided into three equally important phases: preoperative (before surgery), intra-operative (during surgery), and postoperative (after surgery).

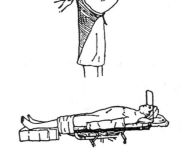

Fig. 12-4　peri-operative nursing

The Pre-operative Stage

The preoperative stage begins when surgery is chosen as the appropriate treatment for a patient and ends when the patient is brought to the operating room. Regardless of whether surgery is major or minor, surgery is a stressor to the body and induces both physiological and psychological stress reactions. Therefore, both physiological and psychological preparation are necessary. Physiological preparation may consist of a complete medical history and physical exam, including the patient's surgical and anesthesia background. Careful and thorough preoperative teaching of patients and their families can be the most important part of the perioperative experience.

The Intra-operative Stage

The intra-operative stage begins with the patient's arrival in the operating room (OP) and ends with the patient's transfer to the recovery room. During surgery (or intraoperatively) the "circulating" nurse and the "scrub" nurse coordinates with the surgeon, anesthesia provider and each other to provide care to the surgical patient in the OP.

The functions of the operating room nurses include: explain all preparation, and answer last-minute questions; ensure proper functioning of equipment and electrical devices, and maintain aseptic technique; verify the patient's identification, verify that the informed consent is signed in the chart; observe the patient for adverse effects of preoperative medications; confirm that both the surgeon and the anesthesiologist are aware of any patient allergies and abnormalities in patient test result.

The Postoperative Stage

The postoperative stage begins as soon as the operation is finished. The goal of postoperative care is to prevent complications such as infection, to promote healing of the surgical incision, and to return the patient to a state of health.

Pain management, which prevent postoperative complications, is the most vital function of the nurse. Assessment includes observing the patient for signs of discomfort including facial bitter, and/or restlessness. Pain medication is administered only according to the doctor's orders and changed according to the patient's response.

Surgical wound sites should be assessed upon receiving the patient. The nurse is responsible for inspection and assessment of proper functioning and maintenance of surgical drains, and drainage on the dressing and the bed underneath the patient. The patient's wound should be inspected for any erythema and warmth (infection) or increases in swelling (hematoma).

Fluid volume deficit and excess are common postoperative complications. Continuous and accurate measurement of intake and output in the postoperative patient is a critical responsibility of the surgical nurse. Comparing intake with output is the best assessment of fluid status. Output should equal about two-thirds of intake over 24 hours.

(451 words)

Words in Focus

peri-operative /ˌpiəriˈɒpərətiv/	adj.	围手术期的
stressor /ˈstresə/	n.	紧张性刺激；应激源
physiological /ˌfiziəˈlɑdʒikəl/	adj.	生理的
psychological /ˌsaikəˈlɑːdʒikl/	adj.	心理的
administer /ədˈministə/	v.	（给予病人）药物
erythema /ˌeriˈθiːmə/	n.	红斑
hematoma /ˌhiːməˈtoumə/	n.	血肿
deficit /ˈdɛfisit/	n.	不足

ER-12-21
扫一扫 读一读

Useful Expressions

medical history	病历；病史
physical exam	体格检查
adverse effect	副作用
pain management	疼痛管理
fluid volume	流体量

ER-12-22
扫一扫 看一看

Post-reading

I. Check your comprehension

I. Choose the best answer to complete each sentence with the information from the text.

1. Peri-operative nursing is focused on care for patients undergoing _____ surgery.

   A. major　　　　　　　B. minor　　　　　　　C. any type of

2. Physiological preparation may consist of a complete medical history and physical exam, including the following except _____.

   A. the patient's surgical background

   B. the patient's anesthesia background

   C. private secret

3. Careful and thorough preoperative teaching of _____ can be the most important part of the peri-operative experience.

   A. patients　　　　　　B. both of them　　　　　C. their families

4. Continuous and accurate measurement of intake and output in the postoperative patient is a _____ responsibility of the surgical nurse.

笔记

A. critical　　　　　　B. useful　　　　　　C. practical

5. Output should equal about _____ of intake over 24 hours.

　　A. two-thirds　　　　B. one fifth　　　　C. one half

II. Vocabulary activities

Find a word or phrase from the box below to complete each sentence. Change word forms where necessary.

assess	administer	be divided into	coordinate with	infection
complication	comfort	focus	psychological	compare

1. Peri-operative nursing is _____ on care for patients undergoing any type of surgery.

2. Peri-operative nursing _____ three equally important phases.

3. A mental disorder is also called a _____ disorder.

4. The data from this study has been used to make a risk _____.

5. Pneumonia is a serious lung _____.

6. During surgery nurses _____ the surgeon, anesthesia provider and each other to provide care to the surgical patient in the OP.

7. Pain medication is _____ only according to the doctor's orders and changed according to the patient's response.

8. Post-operative _____ could occur.

9. Assessment includes observing the patient for signs of _____ including facial bitter, and/or restlessness.

10. _____ intake with output is the best assessment of fluid status.

III. Supplementary

Text B

A fracture is a complete or incomplete break in a bone. Fractures commonly happen because of car accidents, fall or sport injuries. Patients with a fracture require immobilization.

Pre-reading

1. What is the definition of immobilization?

2. What is traction?

Immobilization

Immobilization is the treatment of choice for common musculoskeletal problems. It refers to the process of traction and holding a joint or bone in place with a splint, cast, or brace. Immobilization can help reduce pain, swelling, and muscle spasm.

Traction

Traction is the application of a pulling force to a specific part of the body to straighten broken bones and immobilize fractured bones, relieve muscle spasm, and correct flexion contractures, deformities, and dislocations. To be effective traction, there must be a pull in the opposite direction (counter traction).

Traction can either be applied through the skin (skin traction)

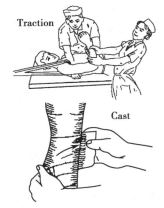

Fig. 12-5　traction & cast

or through pins inserted into bones (skeletal traction).

Nursing care related to traction includes the following:

Assessment of traction:

Frequent checks for the "5Ps" of muscle ischemia: progressive pain, pulselessness, paresthesia, paralysis, pallor.

Frequent neurovascular checks: pulse, nail beds (cyanosis, capillary refill), skin (blanching, coldness, lack of sensation).

Splint, cast or brace

A splint is often used to immobilize a dislocated joint, an injured arm or leg immediately after an injury. It's also often used for finger injuries, such as fractures or baseball finger. Casts are generally used for immobilization of a broken bone. Braces are used to support, align or hold a body part in the correct position, sometimes used after a surgical procedure is performed on an arm or leg. They can also be used for an injury.

Nursing care of the patient with a splint, cast or brace includes:

Checking neurovascular status frequently; Noting color of the skin distal to the affected extremity; Noting drainage, swelling, irritation, odor, or bleeding; Assessing balance and coordination; Assessing the 5Ps of muscle ischemia; Safety and comfort; Emotional support.

After a cast or splint has been put on, the injured arm or leg should be elevated for 24 to 72 hours. It is recommended that the person lie or sit with the injured arm or leg raised above the level of the heart. Fingers or toes can be exercised as much as can be tolerated after casting. This has been found to decrease swelling and prevent stiffness. After the cast, splint, or brace is removed, gradual exercise is usually performed to regain muscle strength and motion.

Normally, the surgical or injured area heals appropriately with the help of immobilization. After immobilization is discontinued, an appropriate rehabilitation program under the supervision of a physical therapist should be carried out to regain range of motion and strength.

(404 words)

Words in Focus

immobilization /iˌmoʊbilaiˈzeiʃn/	*n.*	制动
traction /ˈtrækʃən/	*n.*	牵引
spasm /ˈspæzəm/	*n.*	痉挛；抽搐
splint /splint/	*n.*	（固定骨折的）夹板
cast /kæst/	*n.*	石膏
brace /breis/	*n.*	支持物，支架
paresthesia /ˌpærəsˈθiːʒə/	*n.*	感觉异常
paralysis /pəˈrælisis/	*n.*	麻痹，瘫痪
pallor /ˈpælə/	*n.*	（脸色等的）苍白，灰白
neurovascular /njʊəroʊˈvæskjʊlə(r)/	*adj.*	神经与血管的
distal /ˈdistəl/	*adj.*	末梢的，末端的
ischemia /isˈkiːmiə/	*n.*	局部缺血

Useful Expressions

hold...in place	把……固定就位
flexion contracture	屈曲挛缩
capillary refill time	毛细血管再充盈时间

ER-12-27
扫一扫 读一读

ER-12-28
扫一扫 看一看

笔记

under the supervision of　　　　　　　　　　　　　　在……的监督/指导下

Post-reading

I. Check your comprehension

Answer the following questions with the information from the text.

1.　What are frequent checks for the "5Ps" of muscle ischemia?

_____

_____

2.　What are proper materials for immobilization?

_____

_____

3.　What does nursing care of the patient with a splint, cast or brace include?

_____

_____

4.　What are the suggestions of the doctor after the cast, splint or brace is removed?

_____

_____

II. Vocabulary activities

Find a word or phrase from the box below to complete each sentence. Change word forms where necessary.

surgical	reduce	motion	supervision	specific
immobilize	effect	affect	lie	stiff

1.　Immobilization can help _____ pain, swelling, and muscle spasm.
2.　First-time license holders have to work under _____.
3.　This has been found to decrease swelling and prevent _____.
4.　It is recommended person _____ or sit with the injured arm or leg raised above the level of the heart.
5.　After the cast, splint, or brace is removed, gradual exercise is usually performed to regain muscle strength and _____.
6.　A splint is often used to _____ a dislocated joint, an injured arm or leg immediately after an injury.
7.　To be _____ traction, there must be a pull in the opposite direction (counter traction).
8.　Traction is the application of a pulling force to a _____ part of the body to straighten broken bones.
9.　Noting color of the skin distal to the _____ extremity.
10.The _____ or injured area heals appropriately with the help of immobilization.

III. Supplementary

Part Ⅳ　Writing

Writing a Note of Thanks for Surgery Doctor

　　Doctors are an important part of our society. Although one pays for the services received from a doctor, the life-saving deeds of doctors cannot be measured in terms of money. Gratitude

ER-12-29
扫一扫 答案
"晓"

ER-12-30
扫一扫 练一
练

笔记

towards them can be shown through small acts like thanking them. Even a small thank you note received from a patient would make the doctor feel nice. It would give him/her the satisfaction that his/her work is being acknowledged and appreciated.

Instructions for writing a note of thanks for surgery doctor:

1. Start your letter by reminding the doctor of what he did to earn your appreciation—for example, "Thank you so much for stitching the gash on my son's arm so painlessly."

2. Compliment the doctor on something specific he did during the course of treatment. You might say, for example, "Your gentleness and sense of humor helped ease my son's fear of getting stitches."

3. Acknowledge the team supporting the doctor, if appropriate: "The warm and caring triage nurse set the tone for our whole emergency room stay with her calmness and consideration."

4. End your thank-you note with an upbeat and confident comment on the future, such as "Every time we happen to notice the small scar on my son's arm, we will remember your kindness, skill and good humor."

Examples:

Oct 1ˢᵗ, 2015

Dear Dr.,

/ Name of Doctor /

　　I still remember the day when I was admitted to your hospital for a surgery. It was one of the toughest times in my life. The personal attention and kindness shown by you and your staff helped me overcome my fears about surgery. I have never felt as comfortable going to a hospital in my life before. The counseling I received from you before undergoing the surgery was crucial in my speedy recovery. Thanks a lot!

Sincerely yours,

/ Your Name /

Practice:

　　Nancy White has just undergone a joint replacement surgery, write a letter of thanks for the surgery doctor Dr. Johnson.

_____
_____
_____
_____
_____
_____
_____
_____
_____

ER-12-31
扫一扫 答案
"晓"

Part Ⅴ　Enriching your word power

1.　acr(o)-　　　　　　　　　　　　肢体，表皮
　　acroagnosis /ˈækrəuˌægˈnəusis/　　肢体感觉缺失

笔记

189

acrosclerosis /ˌækrəusklə'rəusis/   肢端硬化病

2.   kinesi(o)-   运动，活动
     kinesioneurosis /kini:ʒn'juərəusis/   运动性神经机能病
     kinesiotherapy /kini:si':əuθerəpi/   运动疗法

3.   arthr(o)-   关节
     arthritis /ɑ:'θraitis/   关节炎
     arthroncus /ɑ:θ'rɒŋkəs/   关节肿大

4.   articul(o)-   关节（坏死）
     articulation /ɑ:ˌtikju'leiʃn/   关节
     articulator /ɑ:'tikjuleitə(r)/   联接器

5.   brachi(o)-   臂
     brachialgia /'breiki:'ældʒiə/   臂神经痛
     brachia /b'reikiə/   臂

6.   cervic(o)-   宫颈
     cervicitis /ˌsɜ:vi'saitis/   子宫颈炎
     cervicodynia /'sɜ:vikɒdiniə/   颈痛

7.   cost(o)-   肋骨，肋
     costopleural /kɒs'təupljuərəl/   肋胸膜的
     costotomy /kɒs'tɔ:təmi/   肋骨切开术

8.   femor(o)-   股骨
     femoral /'femərəl/   股骨的
     femorocele /'femərəsi:l/   股疝

9.   fibr(o)-   纤维
     fibrocalcific /faibrəu'kælsifik/   纤维钙化的
     fibrocartilage /faibrəu'kɑ:tilidʒ/   纤维软骨

10.   my(o)-   肌
     myoatrophy /ˌmaiəu'ætrəfi/   肌萎缩
     myotonia /ˌmaiə'təuniə/   肌强直

11.   radi(o)-   桡
     radial /'reidiəl/   桡骨的
     radiodigital /reidaiəu'didʒitl/   桡骨手指的

12.   ten(o)-; tend(o)-   腱
     tenontagra /tenən'tægrə/   腱痛风
     tendovaginitis /'tendəuvidʒinaitəs/   腱鞘炎

13.   lumb(o)-   腰
     lumboabdominal /lʌm'bəuəbdəminl/   腰腹的
     lumbodynia /lʌ'bɒdiniə/   腰痛

14.   oste(o)-   骨
     osteoporosis /ˌɒstiəupə'rəusis/   骨质疏松症
     osteocachexia /ɒsti:əukæt'ʃeksiə/   骨性恶病质
     osteoarthritis /ɒstiəuɑ:'θraitis/   骨关节炎

15.   vertebr(o)- ; spondyl(o)-   脊椎，脊柱
     spondylexarthrosis /spɒndilik'sɑ:θrəusis/   脊椎脱位

笔记

vertebrae /'vɜ:tibri:/　　　　　　　　　　脊椎

16.　melan(o)-　　　　　　　　　　　　黑

　　　melanin /'melənin/　　　　　　　　黑色素

　　　melanosis /,melə'nəusis/　　　　　黑素沉着病

17.　purpur(o)-　　　　　　　　　　　　紫色

　　　purpura /'pəpjurə/　　　　　　　　紫癜

　　　purpuric /pə'pju:rik/　　　　　　　紫癜的

18.　derm(o)-　　　　　　　　　　　　　皮的，皮肤的

　　　Dermopathy /'dɜ:məupəθi/　　　　皮肤病

　　　dermoplasty /dɜ:'mɒplæsti/ 同 dermatoplasty　　皮成形术，植皮术

19.　dermat(o)-　　　　　　　　　　　　皮的，皮肤的

　　　dermatauxe /dɜ:mə'tɔ:ksi/　　　　皮肤肥厚

　　　dermathemia /dɜ:mət'hi:miə/　　　皮肤充血

20.　hidr(o)-　　　　　　　　　　　　　汗，汗腺

　　　hidroadenoma /hidrəude'nəumə/ 同 hidradenoma　　汗腺腺瘤

　　　hidrosis /hi'drəusis/　　　　　　　发汗，出汗过多

21.　py(o)-　　　　　　　　　　　　　　脓

　　　pyohemia /paiə'ui:miə/ 同 pyemia　　脓毒血症

　　　pyohemothorax /paiəuemʌ'tɔ:ræks/　　脓血胸

22.　myc(o)-　　　　　　　　　　　　　霉菌

　　　mycete /'maisi:t/　　　　　　　　霉菌

　　　mycology /mai'kɒlədʒi/　　　　　真菌学

23.　kerat(o)-　　　　　　　　　　　　角，角膜

　　　keratoderma /kerətəu'dɜ:mə/　　　角皮病

　　　keratitis /,kerə'taitis/　　　　　　角膜炎

24.　seba(o)-　　　　　　　　　　　　皮脂

　　　seborrhagia /si'bɒrhædʒə/　　　　皮脂溢

　　　sebotrophic /sebəu'trəufik/　　　　刺激泌脂的

　　　sebocystomatosis /sebəsistəumə'təusis/　　皮脂囊肿病

Part Ⅵ　Exercise

Directions: *In this section, only one of the following options is correct, please choose.*

（孙　燕　唐瑞娟　吕小君）

ER-12-32
扫一扫 看一看

笔记

Glossary

A

abdomen /ˈæbdəmən/	n.	腹部；腹腔	U5P2C1
abdominal /æbˈdɑ:minl/	adj.	腹部的	U5P3TB
abnormal /æbˈnɔ:ml/	adj.	反常的，异常的	U9P3TB
abnormality /ˌæbnɔ:ˈmæləti/	n.	畸形	U9P2C1
abnormally /æbˈnɔ:məli/	adv.	不正常地	U10P3TB
abscess /ˈæbˈsɛs]	n.	脓肿，脓疮	U4P3TA
absorb /əbˈsɔ:b/	v.	吸收（液体、气体等）	U6P3TA
abulia /əˈbju:lir/	n.	意志缺失	U11P2C2
accelerated /əkˈseləreitid/	v.	加速，促进	U4P3TB
accomplishment /əˈkɑ:mpliʃmənt/	n.	成就，完成，技艺	U11P1PB
Acetaminophen /əˌsi:təˈminəfen/	n.	扑热息痛；对乙酰氨基酚	U9P2C2
achievement /əˈtʃivmənt/	n.	成就，功绩	U11P1PB
acquire /əˈkwair/	v.	学到；获得，取得	U6P3TB
acute /əˈkjut/	adj.	急性的，敏锐的	U4P3TB
adequately /ˌˈædikwətli/	adv.	适当地，充分地	U3P3TB
administer /ædˈministə/	v.	（给予病人）药物	U12P3TA
admission /ædˈmiʃən/	n.	承认；准许进入	U8P2C2
aggravate /ˈægrəvet/	v.	加剧；恶化	U3P2C2
airflow /ˈerflou/	n.	空气流动	U4P2C2
allergy /ˈælərdʒi/	n.	过敏性反应	U6P1PA
alternative /ɔ:lˈtɜ:rnətiv/	adj.	二者择一的	U11P2C1
Alzheimer /ˈɑltshaimər/	n.	阿尔茨海默	U11P2C1
amoxicillin /əmɒksiˈsilin/	n.	羟氨苄青霉素；阿莫西林	U8P1PB
amygdala /əˈmigdələ/	n.	扁桃体结构	U8P2C2
analyze /ˈænəˌlaiz/	vt.	分析；分解；解释	U7P1PA
anaphylactic /ˌænəfiˈlæktik/	adj.	过敏性的	U8P1PA
anemia /ˈɑ:rtəri/	n.	动脉	U3P3TB
anesthesia /ˌænisˈθiʒə/	n.	麻醉	U12P2C1
anesthetic /ˌænisˈθɛtik/	n.	麻醉剂，麻醉药	U5P1PA
anesthetist /əˈnɛsθitist/	n.	麻醉师	U12P2C1
anesthetize /ˈənɛsθiˌtaiz/	v.	使麻醉；使麻木	U5P1PB
aneurysm /ˈænjəˌrizəm/	n.	动脉瘤	U7P3TA
angina /ænˈdʒainə/	n.	心绞痛	U2P2C1
angiotensin /ˌændʒiouˈtensən/	n.	血管紧张素	U3P3TB
anterior /ænˈtiriə(r)/	adj.	位于前部的	U7P3TA
antibiotic /ˌæntibaiˈɑ:tik/	n.	抗生素	U1P2C2
anticonvulsant /ˌæntikənˈvʌlsənt/	n.	抗惊厥的（药物）	U7P1PB
antidepressant /ˌæntidiˈprɛsənt/	n.	抗抑郁药	U11P2C2
antihistamine /ˌæntiˈhistəmin/	n.	抗组织药	U6P1PA
antiviral /ˌæntiˈvairə/	adj.	抗病毒的	U10P3TA
aorta /eiˈɔ:rtə/	n	主动脉	U3P3TA

apex /ˈepɛks/	n.	心尖	U3P3TA
appear /əˈpiə(r)/	v.	出现，显现	U10P3TA
appendicitis /əˌpɛndiˈsaitis/	n.	阑尾炎	U12P2C1
appetite /ˈæpiˌtait/	n.	食欲，胃口	U5P2C2
approach /əˈprəutʃ/	n.	方法；途径；接近	U10P1PA
arbitrarily /ˌɑrbəˈtrɛrəli/	adv.	任意地；武断地	U2P2C2
arrhythmia /əˈriθmir/	n.	心律失常	U3P2C1
artery /ˈɑːrtəri/	n	动脉	U3P3TA
arthritis /ɑːrˈθraitis/	n.	关节炎	U11P3TA
ascites /æˈsaits/	n.	腹水	U5P3TA
aseptic /əˈsɛptik, e-/	adj.	<术>无菌的；经消毒的	U12P1PA
assessment /əˈsɛsmənt/	n.	评估；评价	U1P3TA
asthmatic /æzˈmætik/	adj.	气喘的，似患气喘的	U4P3TB
asymptomatic /ˌesimptəˈmætik/	adj.	无临床症状的	U5P3TA
atria /ˈeitrir/	n.	心房（atrium 的复数）	U3P1PB
atrial /ˈeitriəl/	adj.	心房的	U7P3TA
attach /əˈtætʃ/	v.	把……固定；附上，系	U10P1PA
attitude /ˈætitjuːd/	n.	态度；看法	U10P2C2
auscultation /ˌɔskəlˈteʃən/	n.	听诊	U1P3TB
automatic /ˌɔtəˈmætik/	adj.	自动的	U11P3TB
available /əˈveləbə/	adj.	可获得的；有空的	U1P3TA

B

backflow /ˈbækfloʊ/	n.	回流	U3P3TA
bacteria /bækˈtiriə/	n.	细菌	U4P1PA
bacterial /bækˈtiərirl/	adj.	细菌的；细菌性	U7P2C1
bacteriuria /bækˈtiəriərir/	n.	菌尿	U8P1PB
bathroom /ˈbæθruːm/	n.	厕所；卫生间	U5P2C1
bifocal /ˌbaiˈfoukl/	n.	双光眼镜	U11P1PA
biopsy /ˈbaiɑːpsi/	n.	活组织检查，活体检视	U5P1PA
bladder /ˈblædə/	n.	膀胱	U5P1PB
blameworthy /ˈblemwɜði/	adj.	应受谴责的，该受责备的	U4P3TA
blockage /ˈblɑːkidʒ/	n.	堵塞物，阻塞	U3P3TA
bowel /ˈbauəl/	n.	肠；同情心	U10P2C2
brace /bres/	n.	支持物，支架	U12P3TB
bracelet /ˈbreslit/	n.	手镯	U11P2C1
bradycardia /brædiˈkɑːdir/	n.	心动过缓	U11P2C2
brittleness /ˈbritlnəs/	n.	脆性，脆度；脆弱性	U11P3TA
brochure /ˈbrəuʃə(r)/	n.	小册子，手册	U9P2C1
bronchus /ˈbraŋkəs/	n.	支气管	U4P3TA
bruise /bruz/	n.	瘀伤，青肿；擦伤，伤痕	U6P2C2
bruising /ˈbruːziŋ/	n.	擦伤，挫伤	U5P3TA
burn /bɜːrn/	n.	烧灼疼	U2P2C1
burning /ˈbɜːrniŋ/	adj.	燃烧的	U5P2C1

C

cabinet /ˈkæbinət/	n.	内阁，柜橱	U4P1PA
cachexia /kəˈkeksir/	n.	恶质病	U8P1PA
cadaver /kəˈdævə/	n.	尸体	U8P3TB
caesarean /siˈzeəriən/	n.	剖腹产；<医>剖腹产的	U9P1PB

caffeine /ˈkæfiːn/	n.	咖啡碱；咖啡因；茶精	U9P2C1
calculate	vt.	计算	U9P1PB
calorie /ˈkæləri/	n.	卡路里；大卡	U9P2C1
candidate /ˈkændɪˌdet, -dɪt/	n.	候选人	U6P3TB
capability /ˌkeɪpəˈbɪləti/	n.	能力；才能；才干	U11P1PB
carcinogenic /ˌkɑːrsɪnəˈdʒɛnɪk/	adj.	致癌的，致癌物的	U4P3TB
cardinal /ˈkɑːrdɪnl/	adj.	基本的；最重要的	U1P3TB
cardiopulmonary /ˌkɑːdioʊˈpʌlmənəri/	adj.	心肺的	U2P3TA
caregiver /ˈkerɡɪvə(r)/	n.	照料者，护理者	U11P1PB
carotid /kəˈrɑtɪd/	adj.	颈动脉的	U2P3TA
cartilage /ˈkɑːrtɪlɪdʒ/	n.	软骨	U11P3TA
case /kes/	n.	病案，病例	U12P2C1
cast /kæst/	n.	石膏	U12P3TB
catheterization /kæθɪraɪˈzeɪʃən/	n.	插管术；导尿术	U10P1PA
caution /ˈkɔːʃn/	v.	警告；提醒	U10P1PA
cerebrovascular /ˌserəbroʊˈvæskjələ/	adj.	脑血管的	U7P1PB
certificate /sərˈtɪfɪkət/	n.	证明书	U1P2C2
cervix /ˈsɜːvɪks/	n.	颈部；子宫颈	U9P2C1
characteristics /ˌkærəktəˈrɪstɪk/	n.	特性，特征，特色	U10P3TA
characterized /ˈkærəktəˌraɪzd/	adj.	具有特征的	U5P3TB
chemotherapy /ˌkiːmoʊˈθerəpi/	n.	化疗	U6P2C2
chills /tʃɪl/	n.	寒冷（chill 的名词复数）	U8P2C1
cholesterol /kəˈlestərɔːl/	n.	胆固醇	U3P2C1
chronic /ˈkrɑːnɪk/	adj.	慢性的；长期的	U1P3TA
circulatory /ˈsɜːkjələtɔri/	adj.	循环的	U3P3TA
circumcision /ˌsɜːrkəmˈsɪʒn/	n.	割礼，包皮环切（术）	U6P3TB
cirrhosis /səˈroʊsɪs/	n.	肝硬化；硬变	U5P3TA
claim /kleɪm/	v.	声称；索取	U1P1PA
clinical /ˈklɪnɪkl/	adj.	临床的；诊所的	U10P1PB
clinically /ˈklɪnɪkli/	adv.	临床地	U3P1PB
clip /klɪp/	v.	用别针别在某物上，用夹子夹	U12P1PA
cloudiness /ˈklaʊdɪnəs/	n.	混浊	U12P1PB
collapse /kəˈlæps/	v.	倒塌；崩溃	U2P3TA
colposcopy /ˈkɒlpəskəpi/	n.	阴道镜；阴道窥器检查	U9P3TB
commode /kəˈmoʊd/	n.	便桶；有抽屉的小柜	U2P2C1
compensate /ˈkɑːmpenseɪt/	vi.	偿还，补偿	U11P3TA
complex /kəmˈpleks/	n.	群；复合体	U3P1PB
complexion /kəmˈplɛkʃən/	n.	肤色，面色，气色	U5P2C2
complicated /ˈkɑːmplɪketɪd/	adj.	难懂的，复杂的	U4P3TB
complication /ˌkɑːmplɪˈkeɪʃn/	n.	并发症	U1P3TA
compress /kəmˈprɛs/	vt.	压缩 / 敷布，压布	U11P1PA
compression /kəmˈprɛʃən/	n.	压缩；压紧	U2P3TA
condiment /ˈkɑːndɪmənt/	n.	调味品；佐料	U5P2C2
condition /kənˈdɪʃən/	n.	状态；健康状况	U1P1PB
condom /ˈkɒndɒm/	n.	避孕套，保险套	U9P1PB
confine /kənˈfaɪn/	vt.	限制；局限于	U1P2C1
congenital /kənˈdʒɛnɪtl/	adj.	先天的	U3P1PB
congestive /kənˈdʒɛstɪv/	adj.	充血的，充血性的	U3P3TB
conjunctiva /ˌkɒndʒʌŋkˈtaɪvə/	n.	（眼球）结膜	U5P3TA
conscious /ˈkɑːnʃəs/	adj.	有意识的；神志清醒的	U2P3TA

consciousness /ˈkɑːʃəsnəs/	n.	知觉；感觉	U12P2C2
considerate /kənˈsidərit/	adj.	体贴的；深思熟虑的	U1P2C1
consistency /kənˈsistənsi/	n.	浓度；一致性	U1P3TB
consistently /kənˈsistəntli/	adv.	一贯地，始终如一地	U11P3TA
consultation /ˌkɒnslˈteiʃn/	n.	会诊；请教，咨询	U11P2C2
consumption /kənˈsʌmpʃən/	n.	消费；肺病；耗尽	U2P2C1
contaminate /kənˈtæmə,net/	v.	污染	U6P3TB
contamination /kən,tæməˈneʃən/	n.	污染	U12P1PA
content /ˈkɒntent/	n.	内容；满足；容量	U10P2C2
continuity /ˌkɑːntəˈnuːəti/	n.	连续性；连贯，不间断	U2P1PA
contraception /ˌkɒntrəˈsepʃn/	n.	避孕；节育	U9P1PB
contraction /kənˈtrækʃ(ə)n/	n.	子宫收缩	U9P1PB
conventional /kənˈvenʃənl/	adj.	平常的；依照惯例的	U10P3TB
correlation /ˌkɔrəˈleʃən/	n.	相关，关联	U4P3TA
cough /kɔːf/	n.	咳嗽	U1P1PB
cramps /kræmp/	n.	痛性痉挛，抽筋	U9P2C2
crutch /krʌtʃ/	n.	拐杖，支器	U11P3TB
curable /ˈkjurəbl/	adj.	可治愈的	U4P2C2
cure /kjuə(r)/	v.	治愈；矫正	U10P3TB
currently /ˈkɜːrəntli/	adv.	当前，目前	U6P1PA
curvature /ˈkɜːrvətʃə(r)/	n.	弯曲	U11P3TA
cyanosis /ˌsaiəˈnosis/	n.	苍白病，黄萎病	U4P3TB

D

decline /diˈklain/	n.	减退期，衰退	U11P3TA
decubitus /diˈkjuːbətəs/	n.	卧位；卧姿	U8P3TB
defecate /ˈdefəkeit/	v.	排便；澄清	U10P2C2
defect /ˈdiːfekt/	n.	毛病；欠缺，缺点	U10P1PB
deficiency /diˈfiʃənsi/	n.	缺乏；缺点，缺陷	U6P3TB
deficit /ˈdɛfisit/	n.	不足	U12P3TA
deformity /diˈfɔːrməti/	n.	残缺，残废，畸形的人或物	U11P1PA
degenerate /diˈdʒenəreit/	vi./adj.	退化 / 退化的	U11P3TA
degeneration /di,dʒenəˈreiʃn/	n.	变性，退化，变质	U11P3TA
degenerative /diˈdʒɛnərətiv/	adj.	退步的，变质的，退化的	U11P3TA
delay /diˈlei/	v.	耽搁；延期；推迟	U10P2C2
deleterious /ˌdeləˈtiriəs/	adj.	有害的；有毒的	U5P3TB
delivery	n.	分娩	U9P1PB
dementia /diˈmɛnʃə/	n.	痴呆	U11P2C1
density /ˈdɛnsiti/	n.	密度	U11P3TA
denture /ˈdɛntʃə/	n.	（一副）假牙；托牙	U7P1PA
dependency /diˈpendənsi/	n.	依赖	U2P3TB
depolarization /diːˈpoulərəˈzeiʃən/	n.	去极化	U3P1PB
depression /diˈprɛʃən/	n.	抑郁（症）	U11P2C2
desensitization /ˌdiːˌsensətaiˈzeiʃn/	n.	脱敏；脱敏作用	U6P1PA
desirable /diˈzairəbəl/	adj.	可取的；令人满意的	U2P3TB
detect /diˈtekt/	vt.	查明	U9P3TA
deterioration /di,tiəriəˈreiʃn/	n.	恶化；退化	U8P3TA
diabetes /ˌdaiəˈbitis, -tiz/	n.	糖尿病；多尿症	U8P3TA
diabetic /ˌdaiəˈbɛtik/	adj.	糖尿病的	U6P2C1
diagnose /ˌdaiəgˈnous/	v.	诊断；判断	U6P2C1

diagnosis /ˌdaiəgˈnousis/	n.	诊断	U1P2C1
diagnostic /ˌdaiəgˈnɑːstik/	adj.	诊断的；判断的	U7P1PA
dialysis /ˌdaiˈæləsis/	n.	透析	U8P3TA
diaphragm /ˈdaiəfræm/	n.	避孕环	U9P1PB
diaphragm /ˈdaiəˌfræm/	n.	横膈膜	U3P3TA
diaphragmatic /daiəfrægˈmætik/	adj.	横膈膜的	U1P3TB
diarrhea /ˌdaiəˈriə/	n.	腹泻；痢疾	U3P2C2
digest /daiˈdʒest/	v.	消化；吸收	U10P2C2
digestible /daiˈdʒɛstəbəl, di-/	adj.	易消化的	U5P2C2
dilation /daiˈleiʃn/	n.	膨胀，扩张，扩大	U4P2C2
dilator /daiˈleitə/	n.	（外科用的）扩张器	U9P2C2
disability /ˌdisəˈbiliti/	n.	残疾；无力	U7P3TA
discharge /disˈtʃɑːdʒ/	vi.	出院	U1P2C2
discoloration /disˌkʌləˈreʃən/	n.	变色，褪色	U12P1PB
discontinue /ˌdiskənˈtinju/	v.	（使）终止，中断，中止	U7P1PB
disfunction /disˈfʌŋkʃən/	n.	机能不良，功能紊乱	U11P3TA
dishearten /disˈhɑːrtn/	v.	使失去勇气，使失去信心	U2P2C2
dislocation /ˌdisləˈkeiʃən/	n.	脱位	U11P3TB
dispense /diˈspɛns/	v.	分配，分给	U2P3TB
distal /ˈdistəl/	adj.	末梢的，末端的	U12P3TB
disturbance /diˈstɜːrbəns/	n.	困扰；打扰	U1P3TA
dizzy /ˈdizi/	adj.	晕的	U3P1PA
document /ˈdɑːkjumənt/	v.	记录；证明	U2P1PA
donor /ˈdounə(r)/	n.	捐赠者；供血者	U8P3TB
dopamine /ˈdoupəmiːn/	n.	<生化> 多巴胺	U7P3TB
dosage /ˈdəusidʒ/	n.	（药物等的）剂量；服法	U10P2C2
dose /dous/	n.	剂量，药量	U2P3TB
drastically /ˈdrɑːstikli/	adv.	大大地，彻底地	U9P3TB
drowsy /ˈdrauzi/	adj.	昏昏欲睡的；沉寂的	U5P1PA
dynamic /daiˈnæmik/	adj.	动态的；不断变化的	U1P3TA
dyspnea /dispˈniə/	n.	呼吸困难	U4P3TB
dysuria /disˈjuriə/	n.	排尿困难	U8P2C1

E

eclampsia /iˈklæmpsiə/	n.	子痫惊厥	U9P3TA
edema /iˈdiːmə/	n.	浮肿；水肿	U8P2C2
effective /fektiv/	adj.	有效的；起作用的	U10P2C1
effectiveness /əˈfɛktivnis/	n.	作用；效应；效果	U2P1PA
elasticity /ilæˈstisiti/	n.	弹性	U11P3TA
elderly /ˈeldərli/	n.	老年人	U11P1PA
electrocardiogram /iˌlektrouˈkɑːrdiougræm/	n.	心电图	U3P1PB
electrode /iˈlektroud/	n.	电极；电焊条	U7P3TB
electroencephalography /iˈlektrouensefəˈlɒgrəfi/	n.	脑电图学，脑电描记法	U7P1PB
elicit /iˈlisit/	vt.	引起；引出	U1P3TB
eliminate /iˈliməˌnet/	vt.	淘汰；排除	U8P3TB
embarrassing /imˈbærəsiŋ/	adj.	使人尴尬的；令人为难的	U2P2C1
emergency /iˈmɜːrdʒənsi/	n.	紧急情况；突发事件	U2P3TA
emphysema /ˈemfiˈsiːmə/	n.	肺气肿	U4P2C2
endoscope /ˈendəskoup/	n.	内窥镜	U5P1PA
endoscopy /enˈdɑːskəpi/	n.	内窥镜检查术	U5P1PB

enteral /'entərəl/	adj.	肠的	U2P3TB
enzymes /'enzaim/	n.	酶	U5P3TB
epilepsy /'epilepsi/	n.	癫痫，羊癫疯	U7P1PB
episodes /'episoudz/	n.	插曲，片断	U5P3TB
equilibrium /,ikwə'libriəm/	n.	平衡，平静	U11P3TA
erythema /,eri'θi:mə/	n.	红斑	U12P3TA
evaluate /i'vælju,et/	vt.	评价；对……评价	U1P3TA
eventually /i'ventʃuəli/	adv.	终究；终于，最后	U9P3TB
evidence /'evidəns/	n.	证据；迹象；明显	U10P3TA
exertion /ig'zɜ:rʃn/	n.	费力；劳累	U2P2C1
expectorate /ik'spɛktəret/	v.	咳出，吐痰	U4P1PA
exposure /ik'spouʒə(r)/	n.	暴露	U6P3TB
eyelids /'ailids/	n.	眼睑	U8P2C2

F

falling /'fɔ:liŋ/	n.	落下，坠落	U11P1PA
fatal /'fetl/	adj.	致命的	U1P3TA
fatigue /fə'tig/	n.	疲乏，杂役	U4P3TB
fatigued /fə'tigd/	adj.	疲乏的	U6P2C2
feverish /'fivəriʃ/	adj.	发热的，极度兴奋的	U4P1PB
fibrillation /,fibrə'leiʃən/	n.	肌纤维震颤	U7P3TA
fibrosis /fai'brousis/	n.	纤维化，纤维症	U5P3TA
file /fail/	n.	档案，文件	U1P1PB
filter /'filtə/	vt.	过滤	U8P3TA
fist /fist/	n.	拳，拳头	U2P2C2
flatulence /'flætʃəns/	n.	胃肠气胀	U6P2C1
flexibility /,flɛksə'biləti/	n.	屈曲性	U11P3TA
flexible /'flɛksəbəl/	adj.	灵活的；柔韧的	U5P1PA
fluid /'fluid/	n.	液体	U6P3TB
fluoroscopic /flu(:)ərə'skɒpik/	adj.	荧光镜的，荧光检查法的	U4P2C1
forgetfulness /fə'getflnəs/	n.	健忘	U11P2C1
fracture /'fræktʃə/	n.	破裂，骨折	U11P1PA
framework /'freimwɜ:rk/	n.	构架；框架	U2P1PA
frequent /'frikwənt/	adj.	频繁的，时常发生的	U6P2C1
furnishing /'fɔniʃiŋ/	n.	家具，设备，陈设品，服饰品	U11P2C1

G

gallbladder /'gɔ:l,blædə/	n.	胆囊	U5P3TB
gallipot /'gæli,pɒt/	n.	陶罐，药罐	U12P1PB
gallstones /'gɔ:lstounz/	n.	胆（结）石	U5P3TB
gastrointestinal /,gæstrouin'testinl/	adj.	胃与肠的	U5P1PB
gastroscopy /gæs'trɒskəpi/	n.	胃镜检查法	U5P1PA
gender /'dʒɛndə/	n.	性别	U7P3TB
gestation /dʒe'steiʃn/	n.	怀孕；怀孕期	U9P2C1
ginseng /'dʒin,sɛŋ/	n.	人参	U8P3TB
glucose /'glu:kous/	n.	葡萄糖，右旋糖	U6P2C1
glycogen /'glaikoudʒən/	n.	糖原	U11P3TA

H

hairpin /'herpin/	n.	发夹	U7P1PA

hazard /'hæzərd/	n.	危险；冒险的事	U7P2C2
heal /hi:l/	v.	（使）康复，复原	U12P2C2
helmet/'hɛlmit/	n.	头盔；钢盔	U7P2C2
hematoma /,hi:mə'toumə/	n.	血肿	U12P3TA
hematuria /,hi:mə'tju:riə/	n.	尿血；血尿症	U8P2C2
hemorrhagic /'hemərædʒaik/	adj.	出血性的	U7P3TA
hemostasis /,hi:mə'steisis/	n.	止血；止血法	U8P3TB
hepatitis /,hɛpə'taitis/	n.	肝炎	U5P3TA
herbicide /'ɜ:rbisaid/	n.	除草剂	U7P3TB
hesitate /'heziteit/	vi.	犹豫	U1P2C1
hormones /'hɔ:moun/	n.	荷尔蒙，激素	U5P3TB
hospitalization /,hɑspitli'zeʃən/	n.	住院治疗；送入医院	U7P2C1
hospitalize /'hɒspitəlaiz/	vt.	把……送入医院治疗	U8P3TA
hydronephrosis /,haidrəni'frousis/	n.	肾盂积水	U8P1PA
hypertension /,haipər 'tenʃn/	n.	高血压	U3P1PA
hyperthyrosis /haipəθaiə'rousis/	n.	甲状腺功能亢进	U8P1PA
hypobulia /haipou'bju:liə/	n.	意志薄弱，意志消沉	U11P2C2
hypotension /haipə'tenʃən/	n.	低血压	U8P1PA
hypothyroidism /,haipou'θairɔidizəm/	n.	甲状腺功能减退	U3P3TB

I

ibuprofen /,aibju:'prəufen/	n.	布洛芬，异丁苯丙酸	U9P2C2
iliacfossa /'ili,æk 'fɑsə/	n.	髂窝	U8P3TB
illegible /i'lɛdʒəbəl/	adj.	无法辨认的	U2P3TB
immobilization /i,moubəlai'zeiʃn/	n.	制动	U12P3TB
immune /i'mjoon/	adj.	免疫的；有免疫力的	U6P1PB
implant /im'plænt/	vt.	植入，插入	U7P3TB
implementation /,implimən'teʃən/	n.	实施；贯彻；执行	U2P1PA
improvement /im'pru:vmənt/	n.	改进，改善	U10P2C1
impulse /'im,pʌls/	n.	冲动，搏动	U3P1PB
incision /in'siʒən/	n.	切开；切口	U1P2C2
independence /,indi'pendəns/	n.	独立；自主；自立	U11P1PB
independently /,indi'pɛndəntli/	adv.	独立地，自立地	U11P1PB
index /'in,dɛks/	n.	指数	U8P2C2
induce /in'dju:s/	v.	<医>诱导；引起	U9P1PB
infection /in'fekʃn/	n.	<医>传染，感染	U9P2C1
infectious /in'fekʃəs/	adj.	传染的；有传染性的	U10P3TA
inflammation /,inflə'meʃən/	n.	炎症；燃烧	U5P3TA
inflammatory /in'flæmətɔ:ri/	adj.	炎性的，发炎的	U6P1PB
inhalation /,inhə'leiʃn/	n.	吸入；吸入剂，吸入物	U10P1PB
inherit /in'herit/	v.	继承；继任	U10P3TB
initial /i'niʃəl/	adj.	最初的；开始的	U1P3TA
injection /in'dʒɛkʃən/	n.	注射；注射剂	U5P1PA
inpatient /'in,peʃənt/	n.	住院病人	U1P2C1
insert /in'sɜ:t/	vt.	插入；嵌入	U9P2C2
inspect /in'spɛkt/	v.	检查；视察	U1P3TB
instrument /'instrəmənt/	n.	仪器	U5P1PB
insulin /'insəlin/	n.	胰岛素	U6P3TA
insurance /in'ʃurəns/	n.	保险费；保险	U1P1PA
integrate /'inti,gret/	adj.	完整的	U12P1PA

integrity /in'tɛgriti/	n.	完整	U6P3TB
interaction /ˌintə'ækʃən/	n.	相互作用	U11P2C2
interfere /ˌintər'fir/	v.	干预,干涉	U6P3TB
interior /in'tiriə(r)/	n.	内部;内心	U5P1PB
intervene /ˌintər'vi:n/	vi.	干预;阻碍	U1P3TA
intervention /ˌintə'venʃn/	n.	干预,介入	U3P3TB
intestines /in'testinz/	n.	肠	U5P2C1
intracerebral /ˌintrəsə'ri:brəl/	adj.	大脑内的	U7P3TA
intravenous /ˌintrə'vi:nəs/	adj.	进入静脉的,静脉注射的	U8P1PA
inverse /in'vɜ:rs/	adj.	相反的;逆向的;倒转的	U7P3TB
involvement /in'va:lvmənt/	n.	牵连,参与;加入	U11P2C2
iodine /'aiədi:n/	n.	碘	U8P1PA
irregular /i'regjələ(r)/	adj.	不规则的;无规律的	U10P3TA
irritant /'iritənt/	adj.	刺激的,刺激性的	U4P3TA
irritating /'iriteitiŋ/	adj.	刺激性的	U5P2C2
irritation /ˌiri'teiʃn/	n.	刺激	U9P3TB
ischemia /is'ki:miə/	n.	局部缺血	U12P3TB
ischemic /is'ki:mik/	adj.	缺血性的	U7P3TA
itchy /'itʃi/	adj.	(使)发痒的	U10P3TA

J

jaundice /'dʒɔndis, 'dʒɑn-/	n.	黄疸病	U5P3TA

K

kidney /'kidni/	n.	肾;肾脏	U8P2C1
kindergarten /'kindərgɑ:rtn/	n.	幼儿园;学前班	U2P1PB
kyphosis /kai'fousis/	n.	驼背	U11P3TA

L

laboratory /'læbrətɔ:ri/	n.	实验室	U5P2C1
labour /'leibə/	n.	分娩	U9P1PB
lesion /'liʒən/	n.	损害	U6P3TB
leukemia /lu:'ki:mir/	n.	<医>白血病	U6P2C2
limitation /ˌlimi'teʃən/	n.	限制,局限性	U11P1PB
lumbago /lʌm'beigəu/	n.	背痛	U8P2C1

M

macrophage /'mækrə'fedʒ/	n.	巨噬细胞,大噬细胞	U4P3TB
malaise /mæ'lez, -'lɛz/	n.	萎靡不振;不适,不舒服	U5P3TA
malformation /ˌmælfɔ:r'meiʃn/	n.	畸形	U8P1PA
malignant /mə'lignənt/	adj.	恶性的,有害的	U4P3TA
marrow /'mærou/	n.	骨髓;脊髓	U6P2C2
maternal /mə't3:n(ə)l/	adj.	母亲的	U9P3TA
measurable /'mɛʒərəbəl/	adj.	可量度的;可测量的	U2P1PA
mediastinum /ˌmi:diæs'tainəm/	n.	纵隔	U3P3TA
membrane /'mɛm,bren/	n.	隔膜;薄膜	U5P3TA
meningitis /ˌmɛnin'dʒaitis/	n.	脑膜炎	U7P2C1
menopause /'mɛnə'pɔz/	n.	绝经期,更年期	U11P3TA
menstrual /'menstruəl/	adj.	月经的	U9P1PA
metabolic /ˌmetə'bɒlik/	adj.	新陈代谢的;变化的	U3P1PA

metabolism /mi'tæbə,lizəm/	n.	新陈代谢；代谢作用	U5P3TB
microbial /mai'kroubirl/	adj.	微生物的，由细菌引起的	U12P1PA
microorganism /,maikro'ɔrgə,nizəm/	n.	微生物	U6P1PB
micturition /,miktjʊ'riʃn/	n.	排尿	U8P1PB
mifepristone /maifpris'təun/	n.	米非司酮（一种堕胎药）	U9P2C2
milieu /mi:'ljə/	n.	环境	U11P2C2
miscarriage /'miskæridʒ/	n.	流产，早产	U9P1PB
misoprostol /misɒp'rɒztl/	n.	米索前列醇	U9P2C2
mobility /moʊ'biləti/	n.	可动性，移动性	U11P3TB
modality /moʊ'dæləti/	n.	方式，形式，模式	U5P3TB
moderate /'mɑ:dərət/	adj.	中等的；有节制的	U3P3TB
modification /,mɑ:difi'keiʃn/	n.	修改，修正	U6P3TA
morbidity /mɔ:'bidəti/	n.	发病率	U9P3TA
mortality /mɔr'tæləti/	n.	死亡率，必死性	U4P3TA
movement /'mu:vmənt/	n.	运动；活动	U10P2C2
mucous /'mjukəs/	adj.	黏液的，黏液覆盖的	U5P3TA
mucus /'mjukəs/	n.	黏液	U4P2C2
multiple /'mʌltəpəl/	adj.	多重的；多个的；复杂的	U7P1PA
musculoskeletal /,mʌskjəlou'skelətəl/	adj.	肌（与）骨骼的	U11P3TA
mutate /'mju:teit/	v.	变异	U6P3TB
myocarditis /,maiouka:'daitis/	n.	心肌炎	U3P2C2

N

narcotic /nɑ:'kɒtik/	n./adj.	麻醉药／麻醉的	U11P3TB
nauseous /'nɔ:ʃəs/	adj.	感到恶心的	U3P2C1
navigate /'nævi'get/	vt.	横渡，跨越	U11P3TB
nebulization /,nebjʊlai'zeiʃən/	n.	喷雾疗法，喷雾作用	U10P2C1
necklace /'nɛklis/	n.	项链	U11P2C1
neonate /'ni:əuneit/	n.	新生儿	U10P1PA
neurological /,nʊrə'la:dʒikl/	adj.	神经学的；神经病学的	U7P2C1
neurologist /nʊ'ra:lədʒist/	n.	<医>神经病学家	U7P3TB
neurovascular /njʊərou'væskjʊlə(r)/	adj.	神经与血管的	U12P3TB
nocturnal /nɑ:k'tɜ:rnl/	adj.	夜的，夜间的	U6P3TA
normal /'nɔ:ml/	adj.	正常的；标准的	U10P3TA
nourishing /'nʌriʃiŋ/	adj.	有营养的；滋养多的	U8P3TB
noxious /'nɑ:kʃəs/	adj.	有害的；有毒的	U2P3TB
NPO（拉丁语）nil per os	n.	禁饮食	U12P2C1
numb /nʌm/	adj.	麻木的，失去感觉的	U9P2C2
numbness /'nʌmnis/	n.	麻木	U8P1PA
nutritious /nu'triʃəs/	adj.	有营养的；滋养的	U1P2C2

O

obesity /o'bisiti/	n.	肥胖症，肥胖	U3P3TB
objective /əb'dʒɛktiv/	adj.	客观的；目标的	U1P3TA
observe /əb'zɜ:rv/	v.	观察	U1P3TA
occupation /ɑ:kju'peiʃn/	n.	职业；工作	U2P1PB
oestrogen /'ɛstrədʒən/	n.	雌激素	U11P3TA
on-going /'əng'ouiŋ/	adv.	继续存在；不间断地	U11P2C1
optimal /'ɑ:ptiməl/	adj.	最佳的，最优的；最理想的	U7P1PB
optimistic /,ɒpti'mistik/	adj.	乐观的	U11P2C2

optimize /ˈɒptimaiz/	v.	使最优化，使尽可能有效	U10P3TB
organism /ˈɔːrɡənizəm/	n.	有机体；生物体；微生物	U7P2C1
orthopaedic /ˌɔːθəˈpiːdik/	adj.	整形外科的	U11P3TB
orthopedist /ɔːθəˈpiːdist/	n.	骨科医生；整形外科医师	U2P1PB
osteoarthritis /ˌɑːstiouɑːrˈθraitis/	n.	骨关节炎	U11P3TA
osteoporosis /ˌɑːstioupəˈrousis/	n.	骨质疏松症	U11P3TA
overestimate /ˌəuvərˈestimeit/	vt.	对（数量）估计过高	U9P2C1
overlap /ˌouvərˈlæp/	v.	重叠，相交	U3P3TA
overload /ˌouvərˈloud/	n.	过多，过量；超负荷	U2P2C2
overreact /ˌouvəriˈækt/	v.	反应过火	U6P1PB
oxygen /ˈɑːksidʒən/	n.	氧；氧气	U2P2C1
oxygenated /ˈɒksidʒəneitid/	adj.	含氧的	U3P3TA
oxytocin /ˌɒksiˈtəusin/	n.	催产素	U9P1PB

P

pad/pæd/	vt.	给……装衬垫	U7P2C2
painkiller /ˈpenˌkilə(r)/	n.	止痛药	U12P2C2
pallor /ˈpælə/	n.	（脸色等的）苍白，灰白	U12P3TB
palpate /pælˈpeit/	v.	触诊	U2P3TA
palpation /pælˈpeiʃn/	n.	触诊	U1P3TB
palpitation /ˌpælpiˈteʃən/	n.	心悸	U3P2C2
palsy /ˈpɔlzi/	n.	麻痹，中风	U7P3TB
pancreas /ˈpæŋkriəs, ˈpæn-/	n.	胰，胰腺	U5P3TB
pancreatitis /ˌpæŋkriəˈtaitis/	n.	胰腺炎	U5P3TB
papillomavirus /pæpiləuˈmævairəs/	n.	乳头瘤病毒	U9P3TB
paralysis /pəˈrælisis/	n.	麻痹，瘫痪	U12P3TB
parenteral /pəˈrentərəl/	adj.	肠外的	U2P3TB
paresthesia /ˌpærəsˈθiːʒə/	n.	感觉异常	U12P3TB
parturition /ˌpɑːtjuˈriʃn/	n.	生产，分娩	U9P1PB
patent /ˈpætnt/	adj.	专利的；明摆着的	U7P3TA
pathogenic /ˌpæθəˈdʒenik/	adj.	引起疾病的	U4P1PA
pathogens/ˈpæθədʒəns/	n.	病菌，病原体	U4P1PA
pathology /pəˈθɑːlədʒi/	n.	病理（学）	U5P1PA
pavement /ˈpevmənt/	n.	人行道；硬路面	U2P1PB
pedestrian /pəˈdɛstriən/	n.	步行者	U11P1PA
pee /piː/	vi.	小便；撒尿	U8P2C1
penicillin/ˌpɛniˈsilin/	n.	青霉素，盘尼西林	U4P2C1
percussion /pərˈkʌʃn/	n.	叩诊	U1P3TB
perform /pəˈfɔːm/	v.	执行；完成；做；运行	U10P1PA
period /ˈpiəriəd/	n.	时期；（一段）时间	U10P3TA
peri-operative /ˌpiəriˈɒpərətiv/	adj.	围手术期的	U12P3TA
peripheral /pəˈrifərəl/	adj.	外围的，外周的	U3P1PA
persistent /pərˈsistənt/	adj.	持久稳固的	U8P1PB
pesticide /ˈpɛstiˌsaid/	n.	杀虫剂，农药	U7P3TB
pharmacology /ˌfɑːrməˈkɑːlədʒi/	n.	药理学；药物学	U2P3TB
pharmacy /ˈfɑːrməsi/	n.	药房	U1P2C2
phenomenon /fəˈnɑːminən/	n.	现象；事件	U2P2C1
phlegm /flɛm/	n.	痰，黏液	U4P1PB
physician /fiˈziʃən/	n.	内科医生	U1P1PB
physiological /ˌfiziəˈlɑdʒikəl/	adj.	生理的	U12P3TA

physiotherapist /ˌfiziou'θerəpist/	n.	理疗师	U11P3TB
pinch /pintʃ/	v.	捏；挤痛	U2P3TA
placenta /plə'sentə/	n.	胎盘	U9P3TA
pneumoconiosis /ˌnjuməˌkoni'osis/	n.	尘肺病，肺尘埃沉着病	U4P3TB
pneumonectomy /ˌnjumə'nɛktəmi/	n.	肺切除术	U4P3TA
pneumonia /nu'moniə/	n.	肺炎，急性肺炎	U4P1PA
pollen /'pɑːlən/	n.	花粉；＜虫＞粉面	U6P1PA
polyuria /ˌpɒli'jʊrir/	n.	多尿（症）	U6P3TA
porous /'pɔrəs/	adj.	多孔的	U11P3TA
postmature /ˌpəustmətjuə/	n.	过度成熟的（婴儿）；过期产	U9P1PB
postnatal /pəust'neitl/	adj.	出生后的	U9P3TA
postoperative /ˌpəust'ɒpərətiv/	adj.	手术后的	U8P3TB
potential /pə'tɛnʃəl/	adj.	潜在的，有可能的	U6P3TB
precancerous /priː'kænsərəs/	adj.	癌症前期的	U9P3TB
precaution /pri'kɔʃən/	n.	预防措施；预防	U7P2C1
precipitating /pri'sipiteitiŋ/	adj.	促成的，诱因的	U3P3TB
predictable /pri'diktəbl/	adj.	可预知的；可预报的	U11P2C1
preeclampsia /ˌpriːi'klæmpsiːə/	n.	先兆子痫	U9P2C1
pregnancy /'pregnənsi/	n.	怀孕，妊娠	U9P1PA
pregnant /'pregnənt/	adj.	怀孕的	U9P1PA
premature /'premətʃə(r)/	n.	早产儿	U9P1PB
prenatal /ˌpriː'neitl/	adj.	出生前的，胎儿期的	U9P1PA
prescribe /pri'skraib/	vi.	开处方	U1P2C2
prevalence /'prevələns/	n.	（疾病等的）流行程度	U9P3TB
prevent /pri'vent/	v.	预防；阻止；阻碍	U10P2C1
prevention /pri'vɛnʃən/	n.	预防	U2P3TB
prick /prik/	vt.	刺，扎	U7P2C1
primary /'praiməri/	adj.	首要的；主要的	U5P2C2
principle /'prinsəpəl/	n.	原则，原理；准则，道义	U2P3TB
prior /'praiə(r)/	adj.	在……之前；优先的	U10P1PA
procedure /prə'sidʒə/	n.	程序，手续	U6P2C2
product /'prɒdʌkt/	n.	产品；结果	U10P2C1
prominent /'praːminənt/	adj.	突出的，杰出的	U6P3TA
prosector /prə(ʊ)'sektə/	n.	解剖员	U4P3TB
prostate /'praːsteit/	n.	前列腺	U8P3TA
prosthetic /prɑs'θɛtik/	adj.	假体的	U11P3TB
protein /'prouti:n/	n.	蛋白质	U8P3TB
proteinuria /ˌprouti:'nur'i:ə/	n.	蛋白尿	U8P2C2
psychological /ˌsaikə'lɑːdʒikl/	adj.	心理的	U12P3TA
pulmonary /'pʌlməneri/	adj.	肺部的	U11P3TA
pyelography /paiə'lɒgrəfi/	n.	肾盂造影术	U8P1PA
pyelonephritis /paiələuni'fraitis/	n.	肾盂肾炎	U8P2C1

Q

quantity /'kwaːntəti/	n.	量，数量；数目	U6P2C1

R

radiation /ˌredi'eʃən/	n.	放射	U12P2C2
radiologist /ˌreidi'ɑːlədʒist/	n.	放射线技师	U7P1PA
rale /rɑːl/	n.	啰音，水泡音，肺的诊音	U4P2C1

rash /ræʃ/	n.	（皮）疹；爆发		U7P2C1
recipient /ri'sipiənt/	n.	接受者		U8P3TB
recovery /ri'kʌvəri/	n.	恢复；复原		U1P2C1
rectum /'rɛktəm/	n.	直肠		U2P3TB
redden /rɛdn:/	v.	（使）变红		U6P1PB
refer /ri'fɚ/	v.	提到；针对；归因于……		U7P1PA
register /'rɛdʒistə/	v.	登记；注册		U1P1PA
registration /,rɛdʒi'streʃən/	n.	挂号；登记		U1P1PA
regression /ri'grɛʃən/	n.	回到从前；回归；衰退		U2P1PA
regular /'rɛgjələ/	adj.	有规律的；定期的；经常的		U1P2C2
rehabilitation /,rihə'bilə'teʃən/	n.	复原，恢复，康复		U11P3TB
reinforcement /,ri:in'fɔ:rsmənt/	n.	增强，加强		U11P1PB
relative /'rɛlətiv/	n.	亲属；亲戚		U1P2C1
relatively /'rɛlətivli/	adv.	相对地；比较地		U10P1PB
relevant /'rɛləvənt/	adj.	有关的；相关联的		U1P3TA
reliable /ri'laiəbl/	adj.	可靠的		U9P3TB
relieve /ri'liv/	v.	缓解，解除		U3P2C1
remove /ri'mu:v/	vt.	去除		U9P2C2
replacement /ri'plesmənt/	n.	置换		U11P3TB
replication /,rɛpli'keʃən/	n.	复制		U6P3TB
repolarization /ri:,pouləri'zeiʃən/	n.	复极化		U3P1PB
resistance /ri'zistəns/	n.	抵抗；抗力		U10P2C1
respiratory /'rɛspərətɔ:ri/	adj.	呼吸的		U1P3TA
response /ri'spɑ:ns/	n.	反应；回答		U1P3TA
responsible /ri'spɑ:nsəbl/	adj.	负责任的；尽责的		U1P2C1
restriction /ri'strikʃən/	n.	限制，束缚		U3P3TB
resuscitation /ri,sʌsi'teiʃn/	n.	恢复知觉；苏醒		U2P3TA
reversible /ri'vɜ:səbl/	adj.	可逆的；可医治的		U8P3TA
rheumatic /ru'mætik/	adj.	风湿病的		U3P3TB
rigid /'ridʒid/	adj.	僵硬的；严格的		U7P2C1
rimifon /'rimifən/	n.	异烟肼		U4P1PB
routine /ru'tin/	adj.	常规的；例行的		U1P3TB
rupture /'rʌptʃə(r)/	n.	断裂；破裂		U8P3TB

S

saline /'seili:n/	n.	盐水；生理盐水		U12P1PB
sample /'sæmpl/	n.	样品；样本		U8P1PB
sampling /'sæmpliŋ/	n.	抽样，取样		U4P1PA
scalding /'skɔldiŋ/	adj.	滚烫的，灼热的		U8P2C1
scarring /skɑriŋ/	n.	伤疤；瘢痕形成		U5P3TA
schedule /'skedʒu:l/	n.	时刻表，清单，目录		U6P2C1
screening /'skri:niŋ/	n.	筛查		U9P3TB
seafood /'si,fud/	n.	海鲜		U5P2C1
secretion /si'kriʃən/	n.	分泌，分泌物		U4P3TA
sedative /'sɛdətiv/	n.	镇静剂，止痛药		U5P1PA
segment /'sɛgmənt/	n.	分段		U3P1PB
seizure /'siʒə(r)/	n.	捕捉；突然发作		U7P1PB
semen /'simən/	n.	精液		U6P3TB
sensitive /'sɛnsitiv/	adj.	敏感的；感觉的		U6P1PA
sensitivity /'sɛnsə'tivəti/	n.	灵敏性，感光度		U4P1PA

serious /'siəriəs/	adj.	严肃的，严重的；重要的	U10P2C1
severity /sə'vɛriti/	n.	严重，严重程度	U11P1PA
shivery /'ʃivəri/	adj.	颤抖的，发抖的	U4P2C1
shot /ʃɑːt/	n.	注射；发射；企图	U2P2C2
simultaneously /saiməl'teniəsli/	adv.	同时地	U11P3TA
situation /ˌsitʃu'eiʃn/	n.	情况；形势，处境	U10P2C2
smog /smɑːg/	n.	烟雾	U4P3TA
socket /'sɑːkit/	n.	窝，穴，孔	U11P3TB
sodium /'soʊdiəm/	n.	钠	U3P2C1
softly /'sɒftli/	adv.	柔和地；柔软地；温和地	U10P2C1
solution /sə'luːʃn/	n.	溶液；解决	U10P3TA
solvents /'sɒlvənts/	n.	溶剂	U5P3TA
spasm /'spæzəm/	n.	痉挛；抽搐	U12P3TB
specimen /'spɛsəmən/	n.	抽样；样品	U2P2C1
speculum /'spekjələm/	n.	金属镜，诊视器	U9P3TB
spicy /'spaisi/	adj.	辛辣的；有刺激性的	U5P2C1
spine /spain/	n.	脊柱；脊椎	U8P3TA
splint /splint/	n.	（固定骨折的）夹板	U12P3TB
spontaneously /spɔn'teniəsli/	adv.	自然地，自发地	U6P2C2
spur /spə/	n.	骨刺，骨距	U11P3TA
squeeze /skwiz/	v.	压缩；压迫	U2P3TA
standard /'stændərd/	n.	标准规格；标准的	U11P3TB
status /'stetəs/	n.	情形；状态	U1P3TA
sterile /'sterəl/	adj.	无菌的	U12P1PA
sterilize /'stɛrəlaiz/	vt.	消毒；使无菌	U12P1PA
sternum /'stɜːrnəm/	n.	胸骨；胸片	U2P3TA
steroid /'sterɔid/	n.	类固醇	U4P2C2
stethoscope /'steθəskoʊp/	n.	听诊器	U1P3TB
stiff /stif/	adj.	僵硬的	U12P2C2
stillborn /'stilbɔːn/	adj.	死产的；夭折的；流产的	U9P1PB
stimulate /'stimjəˌlet/	vt.	刺激；激励	U1P2C2
stimuli /'stimjəlai/	n.	刺激；刺激物	U1P3TA
sting /stiŋ/	n.	剧痛	U2P2C1
stooped /'stupt/	adj.	弯腰的	U11P3TA
strengthen /'strɛŋkθən,ˈstrɛŋ-,ˈstrɛn-/	vt.	加强，巩固；勉励	U5P2C2
strenuous /'strɛnjuəs/	adj.	紧张的；费力的；热烈的	U5P2C2
streptomycin /ˈstreptə'maisin/	n.	链霉素	U4P2C1
stressor /'stresə/	n.	紧张性刺激；应激源	U12P3TA
stretch /stretʃ/	v.	伸展；延伸	U9P2C2
stroke /strouk/	n.	中风；一击	U7P1PB
struggle /'strʌgəl/	vi.	奋斗，挣扎	U11P2C1
subjective /səb'dʒɛktiv/	adj.	主观的；个人的	U1P3TA
suction /'sʌkʃn/	n.	吸，抽吸	U9P2C2
supervision /ˌsjupə'viʒən/	n.	监督，管理	U11P1PB
supplement /'sʌplimənt/	v.	增补；补充	U10P2C2
support /sə'pɔːt/	v.	支持；支撑；维持	U10P1PB
surgeon /'sɜːrdʒən/	n.	外科医生	U1P1PB
surgery /'sɜːrdʒəri/	n.	外科手术	U5P1PB
surgical /'sɜːrdʒikl/	adj.	外科的；外科手术的	U8P3TB
susceptible /sə'sɛptəbəl/	adj.	易受影响的；易受感染的	U6P1PA

swallow /ˈswɑːloʊ/	v	吞，咽；忍耐，忍受	U5P1PA
sway /sweɪ/	n.	摇摆，摇动	U11P3TA
swell /swɛl/	v.	肿胀	U6P1PB
swelling /ˈswɛliŋ/	n.	膨大，肿胀	U3P3TB
swollen /ˈswoʊlən/	adj.	膨胀的；肿起的	U2P1PB
symbolize /ˈsimbəlaiz/	v.	象征	U3P3TA
symptom /ˈsimtəm, ˈsimp-/	n.	症状；征兆	U1P1PA
symptomatic /ˌsimtəˈmætik, ˌsimp-/	adj.	有症状的	U6P3TA
syndrome /ˈsindrəum/	n.	综合症状；典型表现	U10P3TB
syphilis /ˈsifilis/	n.	梅毒	U9P2C1
systematic /ˌsistəˈmætik/	adj.	系统的；有条不紊的	U2P1PA
systole /ˈsistəli/	n.	收缩	U3P1PB

T

tablet /ˈtæblit/	n.	药片	U8P2C1
tenderness /ˈtɛndənis/	n.	触痛，压痛	U1P3TB
terminate /ˈtɜːmineit/	v.	结束；使终结	U9P1PB
texture /ˈtɛkstʃə/	n.	质地；纹理	U1P3TB
therapeutic /ˌθɛrəˈpjutik/	adj.	治疗（学）的；疗法的	U2P3TB
therapy /ˈθerəpi/	n.	治疗，疗法，疗效	U10P3TA
thick /θik/	adj.	稠密的，不透明的	U4P1PA
thrombectomy /θrɒmˈbektəmi/	n.	血栓切除术	U7P3TA
thrombocytopenia /ˌθrɒmbəˌsaitəˈpiːniːə/	n.	血小板减少（症）	U6P2C2
thromboembolic /ˌθrɒmbouˈembəlik/	n.	血栓栓子的	U7P3TA
thrombolysis /θˈrɒmboulisis/	n.	溶栓	U7P3TA
toxemia /tɒksˈiːmiə/	n.	毒血症；血毒症	U9P3TA
toxic /ˈtɒksik/	adj.	有毒的；中毒的	U8P3TA
traction /ˈtrækʃən/	n.	牵引	U12P3TB
trait /treit/	n.	过多，过量；超负荷	U10P3TB
transfusion /trænsˈfjuʒən/	n.	输液；渗透	U2P2C2
transition /trænˈziʃən/	vi.	转换，过渡，变迁	U11P3TB
transmitted /trænzˈmitid/	v.	传播，发射；传递，传染	U4P1PA
trauma /ˈtrɔːmə/	n.	损伤；创伤；挫折	U10P1PB
treatment /ˈtritmənt/	n.	治疗；处理	U1P2C1
triglyceride /traiˈglisəˌraid/	n.	甘油三酸酯	U5P3TB
trimesters /traiˈmestə(r)/	n.	孕期	U9P1PB
trip /trip/	v.	绊倒；绊	U2P1PB
trolley /ˈtrɑːli/	n.	治疗车	U12P1PA
tuberculosis /tuˈbɜːkjəˈlosis/	n.	肺结核	U4P3TA
tumor /ˈtjuːmə/	n.	瘤	U6P3TB
turbid /ˈtɜːrbid/	adj.	混浊的	U8P2C1
twist /twist/	v.	扭曲；扭转	U2P1PB

U

umbilical /ʌmˈbilikəl/	adj.	脐带的；母系的	U10P1PA
uncurable /ʌnˈkjuərəbl/	adj.	不能治愈的	U11P2C1
underwire /ˈʌndɔ wair/	n.	拉丝；金属网	U7P1PA
undesirable /ˌʌndiˈzairəbəl/	adj.	不良的；不合需要的	U2P3TB
unfasten /ʌnˈfæsn/	vt.	松开；解开	U7P2C2
unintended /ʌninˈtɛndid/	adj.	非故意的；无意识的	U2P3TB

unintentional /ˌʌninˈtɛnʃənəl/	*adj.*	不是故意的；无意的，无心的	U11P1PA
uremia /juˈriːmiə/	*n.*	尿毒症	U8P3TA
urinary /ˈjʊrəneri/	*adj.*	泌尿的；尿的	U8P1PB
urinate /ˈjʊrəneit/	*v.*	排尿；撒尿	U2P2C1
urination /ˌjʊriˈneiʃn/	*n.*	排尿	U8P2C2
urine /ˈjʊərin/	*n.*	尿；小便	U9P1PA
uterus /ˈjuːtərəs/	*n.*	子宫	U9P2C1
utilize /ˈjutlˌaiz/	*v.*	利用，使用	U6P1PB

V

vascular /ˈvæskjələ/	*adj.*	血管的；脉管的	U6P3TA
vein /ven/	*n.*	静脉	U3P3TA
ventilate /ˈventileit/	*v.*	通风；使通风	U10P3TA
ventricle /ˈvɛntrikl/	*n.*	心室，脑室	U4P3TB
ventricular /venˈtrikjələ/	*adj.*	心室的	U3P1PB
viral /ˈvairəl/	*adj.*	病毒的，病毒引起的	U7P2C1
visualize /ˈviʒuəˌlaiz/	*vt.*	使可见	U5P3TB
vital /ˈvaitl/	*adj.*	至关重要的	U6P1PB
vitamin /ˈvaitəmin/	*n.*	维生素	U8P3TB
voltage /ˌkeipəˈbiləti/	*n.*	电位	U3P1PB
vomit /ˈvɑːmit/	*v.*	使呕吐；吐出	U3P2C2

W

walker /ˈwɔːkə(r)/	*n.*	助步架	U11P3TB
wandering /ˈwɒndəriŋ/	*n.*	漫游；流浪；漂泊；精神错乱	U11P2C1
ward /wɔːrd/	*n.*	病房	U1P2C1
weigh /wei/	*v.*	重量为……	U3P1PA
wheeze /wiːz/	*v.*	发出呼哧呼哧的喘息声	U4P2C2
whitish /ˈwaitiʃ/	*adj.*	带白色的，发白的	U4P1PB
womb /wuːm/	*n.*	子宫	U9P2C1

Reference

1. 王文秀，王颖. 护理英语会话. 北京：人民卫生出版社，2011.

2. 雷慧. 实用医院英语. 北京：人民卫生出版社，2011.

3. 徐淑秀，李建群. 实用护理英语. 第3版. 北京：人民军医出版社，2013.

4. 宋军. 护理专业英语. 北京：人民卫生出版社，2006.

5. 刘华平. 国际护士日常英语. 北京：人民卫生出版社，2006.

6. 段功香，李恩华. 护理学基础. 北京：科学出版社，2004.

7. 李树贞，吴嘉中. 护士英语必读. 上海：第二军医大学出版社，1998.

8. 刘文庆，吴国平. 系统解剖学与组织胚胎学. 北京：人民卫生出版社，2004.

9. 徐小贞. 新职业英语. 北京：外语教学与研究出版社，2009.

10. 焦培慧. 医学视听说. 上海：上海交通大学出版社，2013.

11. 陈冬秀. 护理英语. 上海：上海交通大学出版社，2012.

12. 戴月珍. 当代护理英语教程——常见疾病护理. 上海：复旦大学出版社，2011.

13. 护理职业交际英语. 史冬梅. 上海：复旦大学出版社，2013.

14. Ian Wood，胡燕平. Health Matters 医护英语. 第2版. 上海：上海外语教育出版社，2014.

15. 孙秀丽，邱尚瑛. 英语应用基础. 北京：人民卫生出版社，2013.

16. 林达，尤亚尔·卡本尼图，浅仓稔生. 临床医护英语. 长春：吉林科学技术出版社，2004.

17. 王小丽. 医学英语教程. 西安：西安交通大学出版社，2010.

18. 雷慧编. 实用医院英语. 北京：人民卫生出版社，2014.

19. 王文秀，李志红，冯永平. 医务英语会话. 北京：人民卫生出版社，2010.

20. 江晓东. 实用护理英语. 重庆：重庆大学出版社，2008.

21. 桂莉. 考试解析与实战模拟. 上海：上海科学技术出版社，2006.

22. 埃里克·格伦迪宁，罗恩·霍华德. 剑桥医学英语. 北京：人民邮电出版社，2010.

23. 医护英语水平考试办公室. 医护英语水平考试（护理类）考试大纲（第二级）. 北京：高等教育出版社，2010.

24. 刘晨. 涉外护理英语——情景对话2. 北京：外语教学与研究出版社，2011.

25. 张新宇. 妇产科护理学. 北京：人民卫生出版社，2009.

26. 史学敏. 涉外护理英语——阅读与写作1. 北京：外语教学与研究出版社，2007.

27. 胡雁. 儿科护理学（上下册）. 北京：人民卫生出版社，2005.

28. Virginia Allum，Patricia McGarr. 护理英语2. 北京：中国青年出版社，2010.

29. 秦博文. 护理英语综合教程. 北京：人民卫生出版社，2009.

30. 外国护理学校毕业生委员会. 美国CGFNS护士资格考试指南（中英文本）. 第5版. 北京：高等教育出版社，2003.